MEDITERRANEAN
RECIPES

The Certainty of Eating Great Dishes and at the Same Time Improving Your Appearance with Healthy Food

MARCO SALEMI

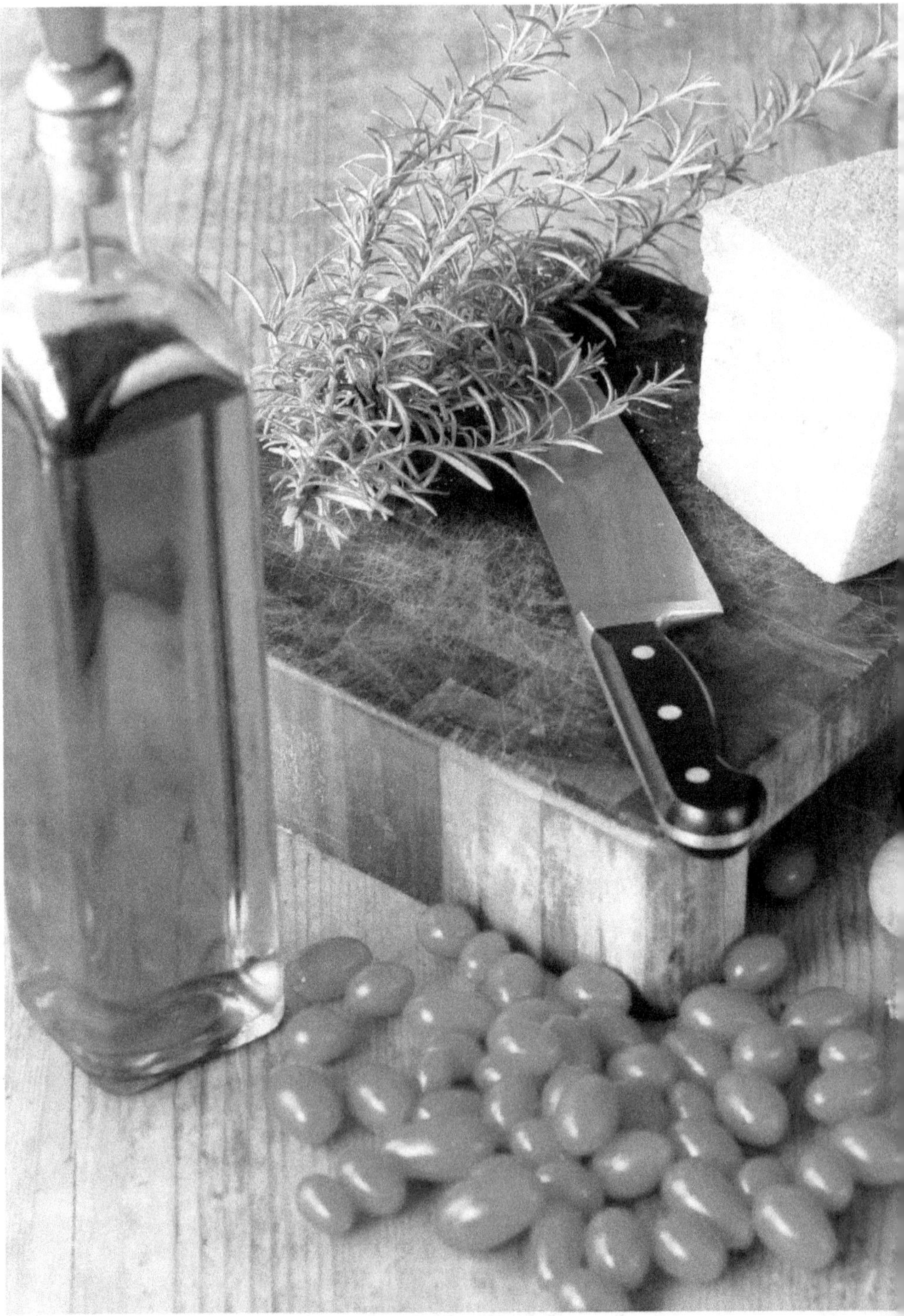

Legal Notice:

Disclaimer Notice:

Table of Contents

Sommario

Introduction

The " Mediterranean diet " can be a generic term that supports the normal eating habits within the countries bordering the Mediterranean. There is no standard Mediterranean diet. A minimum of 16 countries borders the Mediterranean. Eating styles vary between these countries and also between regions within each country due to differences in culture, ethnicity, religion, economy, geography, and agricultural production. However, there are some common factors.

A Mediterranean-style diet typically includes:

lots of fruits, vegetables, bread and other grains, potatoes, beans, nuts, and seeds;
olive oil as the primary source of fat; and
dairy products, eggs, fish, and poultry in low to moderate amounts.
Fish and poultry are used more than meat during this diet. It also focuses on minimally processed plant foods. Wine could also be consumed in low to moderate amounts, usually with meals. Fruit could be a common dessert rather than a sweet treat.

Is the Mediterranean diet a healthy diet to eat?

Year after year, the Mediterranean diet comes out on top of U.S. News and World Report's annual ranking of best diets. A panel of experts judges various popular food plans and diets on criteria including how healthy they are, how well they work, and how easy they are to follow.

The Mediterranean diet is also considered one of the healthiest by many health organizations and dietitians.

So, does it live up to its good reputation?

Does the AHA recommend a Mediterranean-style diet?

Yes. A Mediterranean-style diet can help you achieve the American Heart Association's recommendations for a healthy dietary pattern that:

- emphasizes vegetables, fruits, whole grains, beans, and legumes;

- includes low-fat or fat-free dairy products, fish, poultry, non-tropical vegetable oils and nuts; and

- limits added sugars, sugary drinks, sodium, highly processed foods, refined carbohydrates, saturated fats, and fatty or processed meats.

This type of diet can play a huge role in preventing heart conditions and stroke and reducing risk factors such as obesity, diabetes, high cholesterol, and high vital sign. There is some evidence that a Mediterranean diet rich in virgin vegetable oil can help the body remove excess cholesterol from the arteries and keep blood vessels clear.

What about other popular diets?

You may have heard of popular diets such as paleo, ketogenic (or keto), Atkins, interval, zone, and Whole30. Not all fad diets meet the AHA's science-based criteria for a healthy eating pattern. Some show dramatic results but in the short term and are not heart-healthy.

DASH, or Dietary Methods to Prevent Hypertension, is another eating plan that aligns with AHA recommendations and has been shown to improve health. The DASH diet allows more dairy and meat, while the Mediterranean diet includes regular use of vegetable oil.

A plant-based, vegetarian, or vegan diet can also be a healthy diet to follow.

The most important thing is to focus on the overall quality of your diet, instead of individual nutrients or foods. Try to incorporate more nutrient-dense foods such as vegetables, fruits, legumes, and lean proteins. Limit foods that provide a lot of calories but little nutritional value.

What are the other benefits of a healthy diet?

What you eat affects many aspects of your overall health, including brain health. A healthy diet can improve your ability to think, remember and process information as you age.

In one study, the healthiest consumers at age 50 had a nearly 90 percent lower risk of dementia than those who had the least amount of healthy diets. The Mediterranean and DASH diets have been shown to improve brain health and heart health.

This cookbook offers you a variety of recipes for your Mediterranean diet to follow a healthier and more balanced diet and to improve your energy efficiency and quality of life. Enjoy!

Breakfast

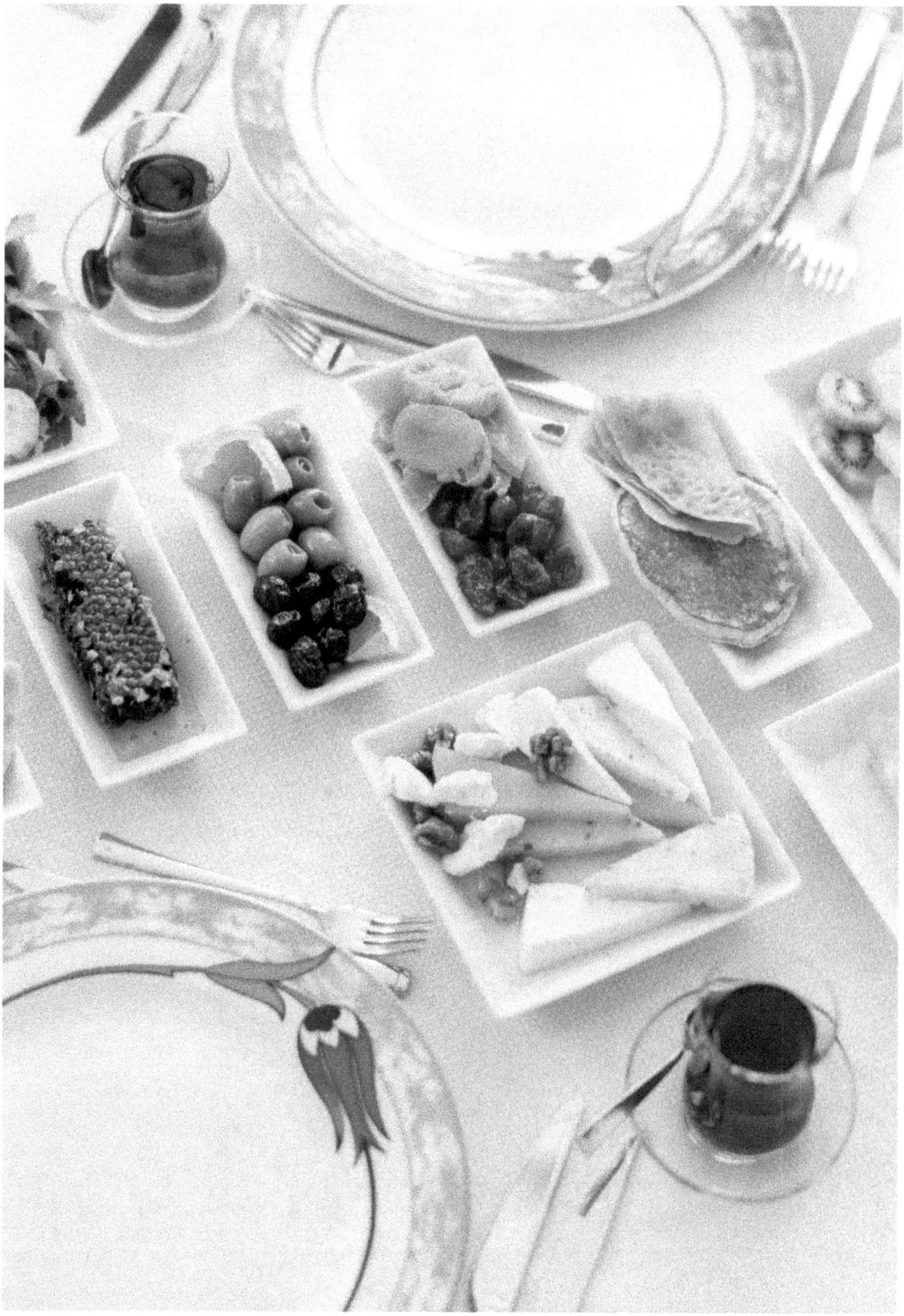

Baked Eggs in Avocado

Prep time: 5 minutes | Cook time: 10 to 15 minutes | Serves 2

Ingredients:
ripe large avocado
large eggs
Salt and freshly ground black pepper, to taste
4 tablespoons jarred pesto, for serving
2 tablespoons chopped tomato, for serving
2 tablespoons crumbled feta cheese, for serving (optional)

Directions:
Preheat the oven to 425°F (220°C).
Slice the avocado in half, remove the pit and scoop out a generous tablespoon of flesh from each half to create a hole big enough to fit an egg.
Transfer the avocado halves (cut-side up) to a baking sheet.
Crack 1 egg into each avocado half and sprinkle with salt and pepper.
Bake in the preheated oven for 10 to 15 minutes, or until the eggs are cooked to your preferred doneness.
Remove the avocado halves from the oven. Scatter each avocado half evenly with the jarred pesto, chopped tomato, and crumbled feta cheese (if desired). Serve immediately.

Per Serving:
calories: 301 | fat: 25.9g | protein: 8.1g | carbs: 9.8g | fiber: 5.0g | sodium: 435mg

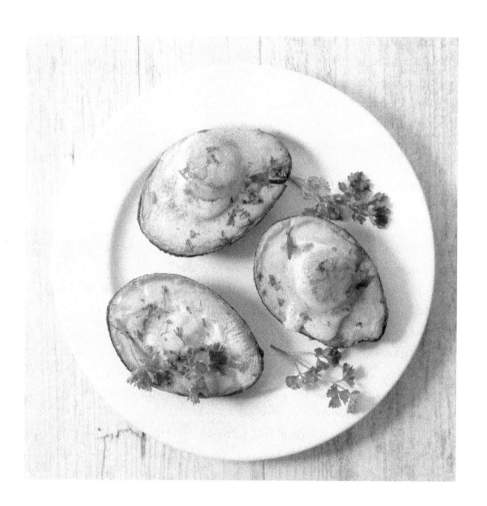

Crustless Tiropita (Greek Cheese Pie)

Prep time: 10 minutes | Cook time: 35 to 40 minutes | Serves 6

Ingredients:
4 tablespoons extra-virgin olive oil, divided
½ cup whole-milk ricotta cheese
1¼ cups crumbled feta cheese
tablespoon chopped fresh dill
tablespoons chopped fresh mint
½ teaspoon lemon zest
¼ teaspoon freshly ground black pepper
2 large eggs
½ teaspoon baking powder

Directions:
Preheat the oven to 350°F (180°C). Coat the bottom and sides of a baking dish with 2 tablespoons of olive oil. Set aside.
Mix together the ricotta and feta cheese in a medium bowl and stir with a fork until well combined. Add the dill, mint, lemon zest, and black pepper and mix well.
In a separate bowl, whisk together the eggs and baking powder. Pour the whisked eggs into the bowl of cheese mixture. Blend well.
Slowly pour the mixture into the coated baking dish and drizzle with the remaining 2 tablespoons of olive oil.
Bake in the preheated oven for about 35 to 40 minutes, or until the pie is browned around the edges and cooked through.
Cool for 5 minutes before slicing into wedges.

Per Serving:
calories: 181 | fat: 16.6g | protein: 7.0g | carbs: 1.8g | fiber: 0g | sodium: 321mg

Buckwheat Porridge

Prep time: 5 minutes | Cook time: 40 minutes | Serves 4

Ingredients:
3 cups water
2 cups raw buckwheat groats
Pinch sea salt
1 cup unsweetened almond milk

Directions:
In a medium saucepan, add the water, buckwheat groats, and sea salt and bring to a boil over medium-high heat.
Once it starts to boil, reduce the heat to low. Cook for about 20 minutes, stirring occasionally, or until most of the water is absorbed.
Fold in the almond milk and whisk well. Continue cooking for about 15 minutes, or until the buckwheat groats are very softened.
Ladle the porridge into bowls and serve warm.

Per Serving:
calories: 121 | fat: 1.0g | protein: 6.3g | carbs: 21.5g | fiber: 3.0g | sodium: 47mg

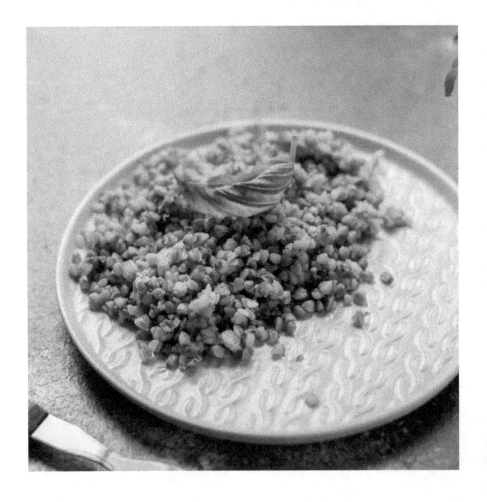

Healthy Chia Pudding

Prep time: 5 minutes | Cook time: 0 minutes | Serves 4

Ingredients:
4 cups unsweetened almond milk
¾ cup chia seeds
1 teaspoon ground cinnamon
Pinch sea salt

Directions:
In a medium bowl, whisk together the almond milk, chia seeds, cinnamon, and sea salt until well incorporated.
Cover and transfer to the refrigerator to thicken for about 1 hour, or until a pudding-like texture is achieved.
Serve chilled.

Per Serving:
calories: 236 | fat: 9.8g | protein: 13.1g | carbs: 24.8g | fiber: 11.0g | sodium: 133mg

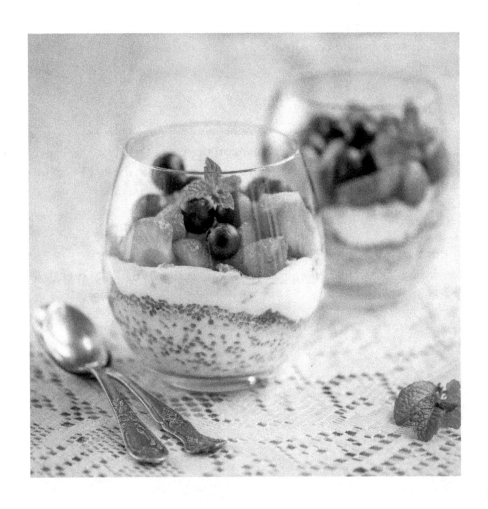

Savory Breakfast Oatmeal

Prep time: 5 minutes | Cook time: 15 minutes | Serves 2

Ingredients:
½ cup steel-cut oats
1 cup water
1 medium cucumber, chopped
1 large tomato, chopped
1 tablespoon olive oil
Pinch freshly grated Parmesan cheese
Sea salt and freshly ground pepper, to taste
Flat-leaf parsley or mint, chopped, for garnish

Directions:
Combine the oats and water in a medium saucepan and bring to a boil over high heat, stirring continuously, or until the water is absorbed, about 15 minutes.
Divide the oatmeal between 2 bowls and scatter the tomato and cucumber on top. Drizzle with the olive oil and sprinkle with the Parmesan cheese.
Season with salt and pepper to taste. Serve garnished with the parsley.

Per Serving:
calories: 197| fat: 8.9g | protein: 6.3g | carbs: 23.1g | fiber: 6.4g | sodium: 27mg

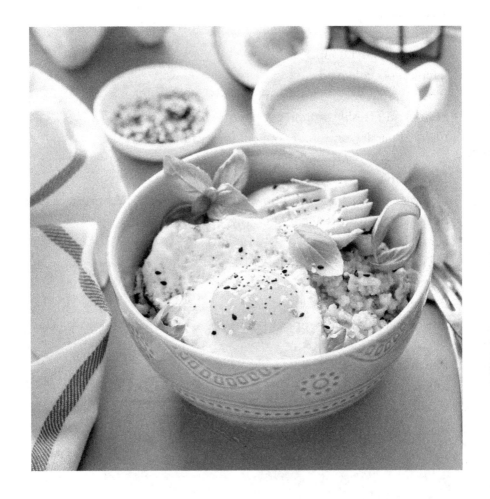

Feta and Olive Scrambled Eggs

Prep time: 5 minutes | Cook time: 5 minutes | Serves 2

Ingredients:
4 large eggs
1 tablespoon unsweetened almond milk
Sea salt and freshly ground pepper, to taste
1 tablespoon olive oil
¼ cup crumbled feta cheese
10 Kalamata olives, pitted and sliced
Small bunch fresh mint, chopped, for garnish

Directions:
Beat the eggs in a bowl until just combined. Add the milk and a pinch of sea salt and whisk well.
Heat a medium nonstick skillet over medium-high heat and add the olive oil.
Pour in the egg mixture and stir constantly, or until they just begin to curd and firm up, about 2 minutes. Add the feta cheese and olive slices, and stir until evenly combined. Season to taste with salt and pepper. Divide the mixture between 2 plates and serve garnished with the fresh chopped mint.

Per Serving:
calories: 244 | fat: 21.9g | protein: 8.4g | carbs:3.5g | fiber: 0.6g | sodium: 339mg

Sides, Salads, and Soups

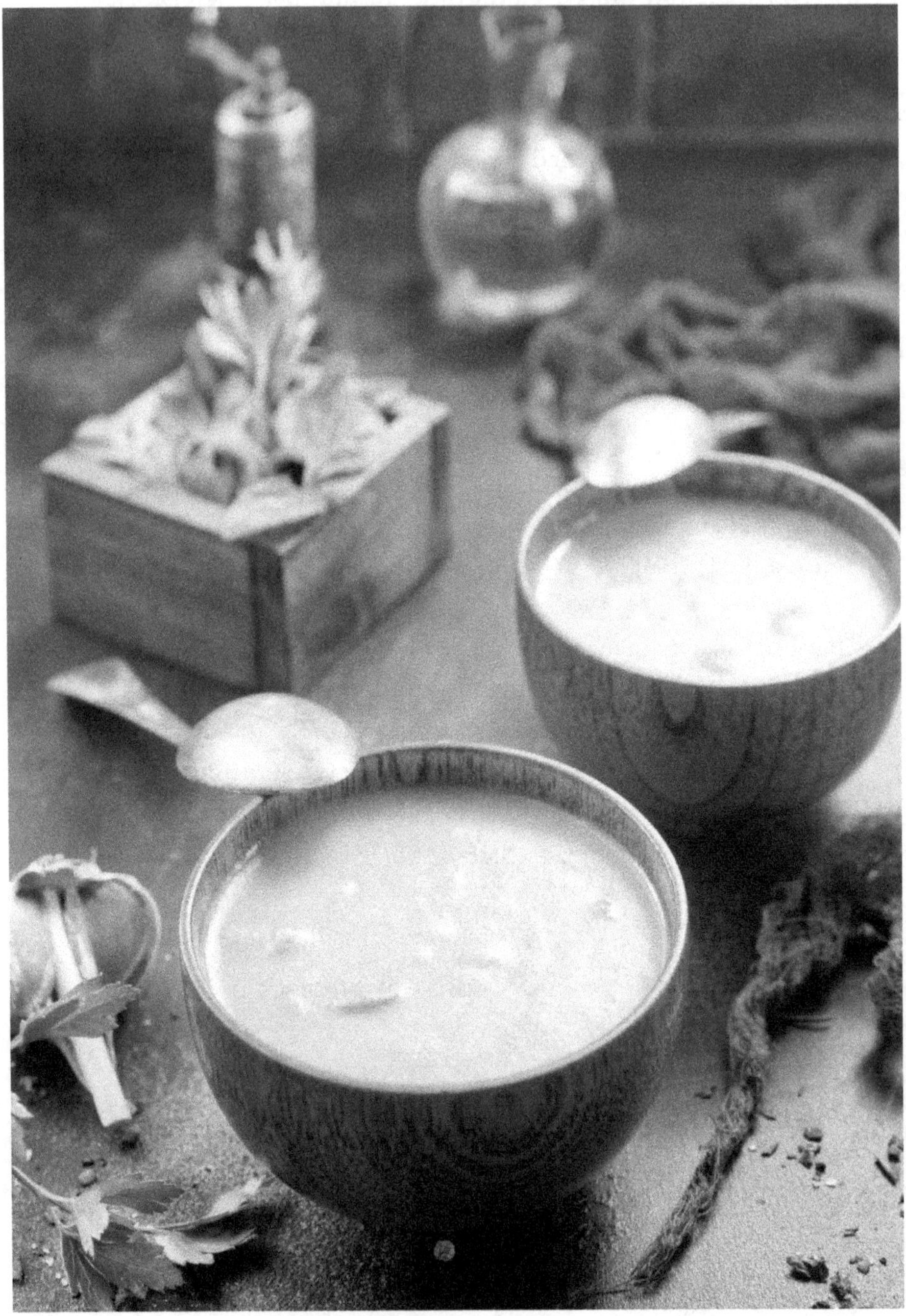

Barley, Parsley, and Pea Salad

Prep time: 10 minutes | Cook time: 10 minutes | Serves 4

Ingredients:
2 cups water
1 cup quick-cooking barley
small bunch flat-leaf parsley, chopped (about 1 to 1½ cups)
cups sugar snap pea pods
Juice of 1 lemon
½ small red onion, diced
2 tablespoons extra-virgin olive oil
Sea salt and freshly ground pepper, to taste

Directions:
Pour the water in a saucepan. Bring to a boil. Add the barley to the saucepan, then put the lid on.
Reduce the heat to low. Simmer the barley for 10 minutes or until the liquid is absorbed, then let sit for 5 minutes.
Open the lid, then transfer the barley in a colander and rinse under cold running water.
Pour the barley in a large salad bowl and add the remaining ingredients. Toss to combine well.
Serve immediately.

Per Serving:
calories: 152 | fat: 7.4g | protein: 3.7g | carbs: 19.3g | fiber: 4.7g| sodium: 20mg

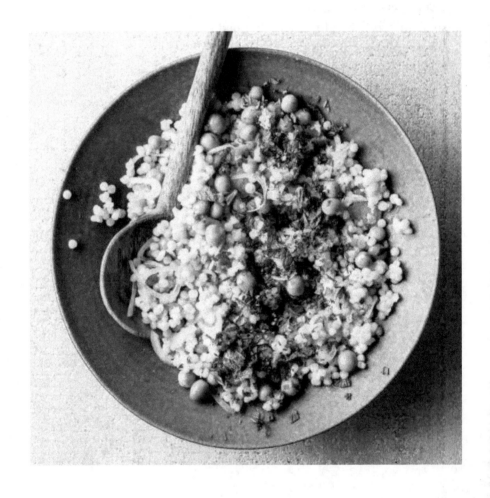

Cheesy Peach and Walnut Salad

Prep time: 10 minutes | Cook time: 0 minutes | Serves 1

Ingredients:
1 ripe peach, pitted and sliced
¼ cup chopped walnuts, toasted
¼ cup shredded Parmesan cheese
1 teaspoon raw honey
Zest of 1 lemon
1 tablespoon chopped fresh mint

Directions:
Combine the peach, walnut, and cheese in a medium bowl, then drizzle with honey. Spread the lemon zest and mint on top. Toss to combine everything well.
Serve immediately.

Per Serving:
calories: 373 | fat: 26.4g | protein: 12.9g | carbs: 27.0g | fiber: 4.7g | sodium: 453mg

Cheesy Roasted Broccolini

Prep time: 5 minutes | Cook time: 10 minutes | Serves 2

Ingredients:
1 bunch broccolini (about 5 ounces / 142 g)
tablespoon olive oil
½ teaspoon garlic powder
¼ teaspoon salt
tablespoons grated Romano cheese

Directions:
Preheat the oven to 400°F (205°C). Line a sheet pan with parchment paper.
Slice the tough ends off the broccolini and put in a medium bowl. Add the olive oil, garlic powder, and salt and toss to coat well. Arrange the broccolini on the prepared sheet pan.
Roast in the preheated oven for 7 minutes, flipping halfway through the cooking time.
Remove the pan from the oven and sprinkle the cheese over the broccolini. Using tongs, carefully flip the broccolini over to coat all sides.
Return to the oven and cook for an additional 2 to 3 minutes, or until the cheese melts and starts to turn golden. Serve warm.

Per Serving:
calories: 114 | fat: 9.0g | protein: 4.0g | carbs: 5.0g | fiber: 2.0g | sodium: 400mg

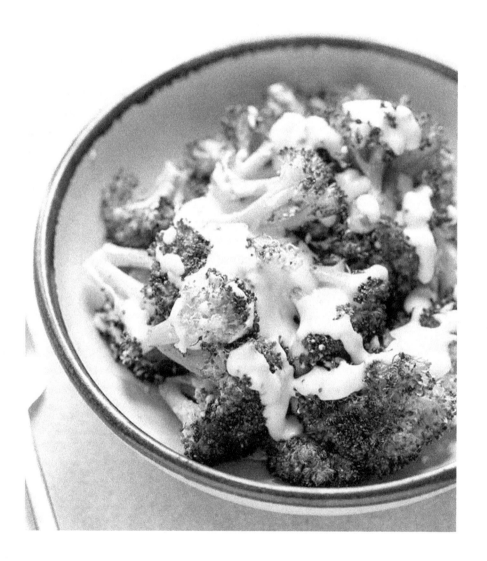

Orange-Honey Glazed Carrots

Prep time: 10 minutes | Cook time: 15 to 20 minutes | Serves 2

Ingredients:
½ pound (227 g) rainbow carrots, peeled
2 tablespoons fresh orange juice
1 tablespoon honey
½ teaspoon coriander
Pinch salt

Directions:
Preheat the oven to 400°F (205°C).
Cut the carrots lengthwise into slices of even thickness and place in a large bowl.
Stir together the orange juice, honey, coriander, and salt in a small bowl. Pour the orange juice mixture over the carrots and toss until well coated.
Spread the carrots in a baking dish in a single layer. Roast for 15 to 20 minutes until fork-tender.
Let cool for 5 minutes before serving.

Per Serving:
calories: 85 | fat: 0g | protein: 1.0g | carbs: 21.0g | fiber: 3.0g | sodium: 156mg

Paella Soup

Prep time: 6 minutes | Cook time: 24 minutes | Serves 6

Ingredients:
2 tablespoons extra-virgin olive oil
cup chopped onion
1½ cups coarsely chopped green bell pepper
1½ cups coarsely chopped red bell pepper
garlic cloves, chopped
1 teaspoon ground turmeric
teaspoon dried thyme
teaspoons smoked paprika
2½ cups uncooked instant brown rice
2 cups low-sodium or no-salt-added chicken broth
2½ cups water
1 cup frozen green peas, thawed
1 (28-ounce / 794-g) can low-sodium or no-salt-added crushed
tomatoes
1 pound (454 g) fresh raw medium shrimp, shells and tails removed

Directions:
In a large stockpot over medium-high heat, heat the oil. Add the onion,
bell peppers, and garlic. Cook for 8 minutes, stirring occasionally. Add
the turmeric, thyme, and smoked paprika, and cook for 2 minutes
more, stirring often. Stir in the rice, broth, and water. Bring to a boil
over high heat. Cover, reduce the heat to medium-low, and cook for 10
minutes. Stir the peas, tomatoes, and shrimp into the soup. Cook for 4
minutes, until the shrimp is cooked, turning from gray to pink and
white. The soup will be very thick, almost like stew, when ready to
serve. Ladle the soup into bowls and serve hot.

Per Serving:
calories: 431 | fat: 5.7g | protein: 26.0g | carbs: 69.1g | fiber: 7.4g |
sodium: 203mg

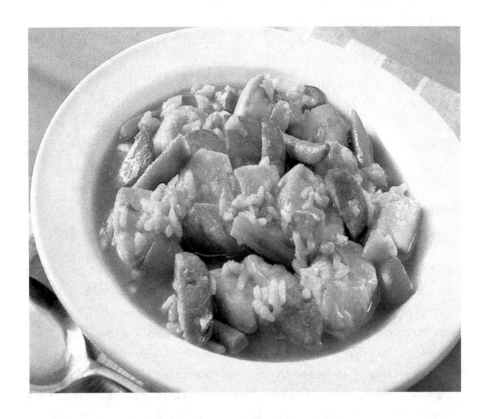

Parmesan Roasted Red Potatoes

Prep time: 10 minutes | Cook time: 55 minutes | Serves 2

Ingredients:

12 ounces (340 g) red potatoes (3 to 4 small potatoes), scrubbed and diced into 1-inch pieces
1 tablespoon olive oil
½ teaspoon garlic powder
¼ teaspoon salt
1 tablespoon grated Parmesan cheese
1 teaspoon minced fresh rosemary (from 1 sprig)

Directions:

Preheat the oven to 425°F (220°C). Line a baking sheet with parchment paper.

In a mixing bowl, combine the potatoes, olive oil, garlic powder, and salt. Toss well to coat.

Lay the potatoes on the parchment paper and roast for 10 minutes.

Flip the potatoes over and roast for another 10 minutes.

Check the potatoes to make sure they are golden brown on the top and bottom. Toss them again, turn the heat down to 350°F (180°C), and roast for 30 minutes more.

When the potatoes are golden brown, scatter the Parmesan cheese over them and toss again. Return to the oven for 3 minutes to melt the cheese.

Remove from the oven and sprinkle with the fresh rosemary before serving.

Per Serving:

calories: 200 | fat: 8.2g | protein: 5.1g | carbs: 30.0g | fiber: 3.2g | sodium: 332mg

Sandwiches, Pizzas, and Wraps

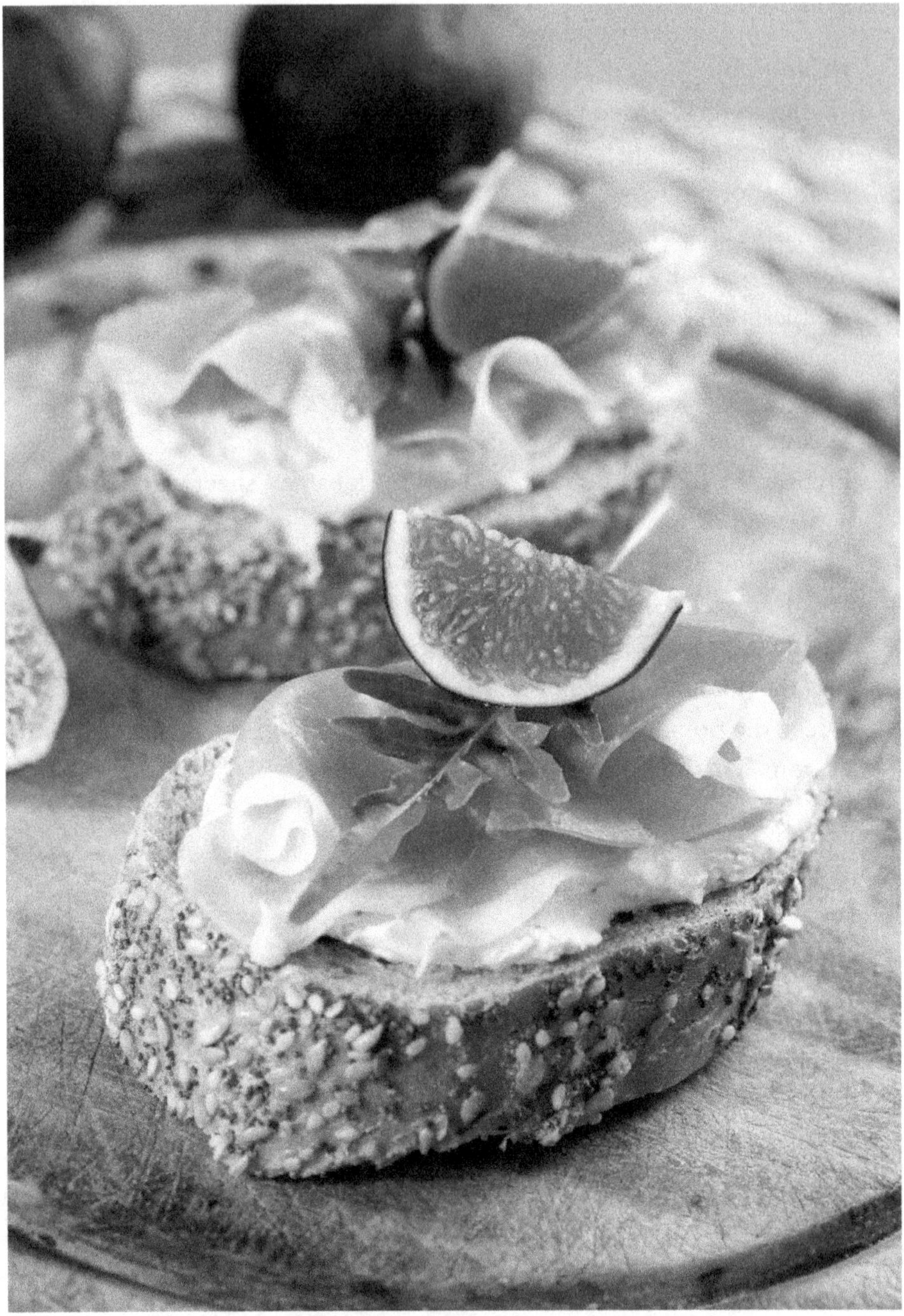

Vegetable and Cheese Lavash Pizza

Prep time: 15 minutes | Cook time: 11 minutes | Serves 4

Ingredients:
2 (12 by 9-inch) lavash breads
2 tablespoons extra-virgin olive oil
10 ounces (284 g) frozen spinach, thawed and squeezed dry
1 cup shredded fontina cheese
1 tomato, cored and cut into ½-inch pieces
½ cup pitted large green olives, chopped
¼ teaspoon red pepper flakes
3 garlic cloves, minced
¼ teaspoon sea salt
¼ teaspoon ground black pepper
½ cup grated Parmesan cheese

Directions:
Preheat oven to 475°F (246°C).
Brush the lavash breads with olive oil, then place them on two baking sheet. Heat in the preheated oven for 4 minutes or until lightly browned. Flip the breads halfway through the cooking time.
Meanwhile, combine the spinach, fontina cheese, tomato pieces, olives, red pepper flakes, garlic, salt, and black pepper in a large bowl. Stir to mix well.
Remove the lavash bread from the oven and sit them on two large plates, spread them with the spinach mixture, then scatter with the Parmesan cheese on top.
Bake in the oven for 7 minutes or until the cheese melts and well browned.
Slice and serve warm.

Per Serving:
calories: 431 | fat: 21.5g | protein: 20.0g | carbs: 38.4g | fiber: 2.5g | sodium: 854mg

---

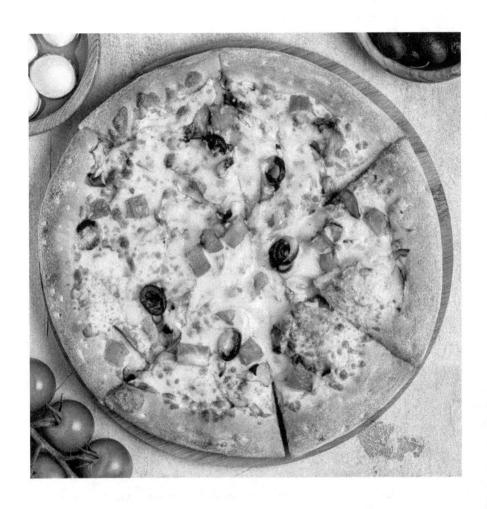

Dulse, Avocado, and Tomato Pitas

Prep time: 10 minutes | Cook time: 30 minutes | Makes 4 pitas

Ingredients:
2 teaspoons coconut oil
½ cup dulse, picked through and separated
Ground black pepper, to taste
2 avocados, sliced
2 tablespoons lime juice
¼ cup chopped cilantro
2 scallions, white and light green parts, sliced
Sea salt, to taste
4 (8-inch) whole wheat pitas, sliced in half
4 cups chopped romaine
4 plum tomatoes, sliced

Directions:
Heat the coconut oil in a nonstick skillet over medium heat until melted.

Add the dulse and sauté for 5 minutes or until crispy. Sprinkle with ground black pepper and turn off the heat. Set aside.

Put the avocado, lime juice, cilantro, and scallions in a food processor and sprinkle with salt and ground black pepper. Pulse to combine well until smooth.

Toast the pitas in a baking pan in the oven for 1 minute until soft. Transfer the pitas to a clean work surface and open. Spread the avocado mixture over the pitas, then top with dulse, romaine, and tomato slices.

Serve immediately.

Per Serving:
calories: 412 | fat: 18.7g | protein: 9.1g | carbs: 56.1g | fiber: 12.5g | sodium: 695mg

Tuna and Olive Salad Sandwiches

Prep time: 10 minutes | Cook time: 0 minutes | Serves 4

Ingredients:
3 tablespoons freshly squeezed lemon juice
2 tablespoons extra-virgin olive oil
garlic clove, minced
½ teaspoon freshly ground black pepper
(5-ounce / 142-g) cans tuna, drained
1 (2.25-ounce / 64-g) can sliced olives, any green or black variety
½ cup chopped fresh fennel, including fronds
8 slices whole-grain crusty bread

Directions:
In a medium bowl, whisk together the lemon juice, oil, garlic, and
pepper. Add the tuna, olives and fennel to the bowl. Using a fork,
separate the tuna into chunks and stir to incorporate all the ingredients.
Divide the tuna salad equally among 4 slices of bread. Top each with
the remaining bread slices.
Let the sandwiches sit for at least 5 minutes so the zesty filling can soak
into the bread before serving.

Per Serving:
calories: 952 | fat: 17.0g | protein: 165.0g | carbs: 37.0g | fiber: 7.0g |
sodium: 2572mg

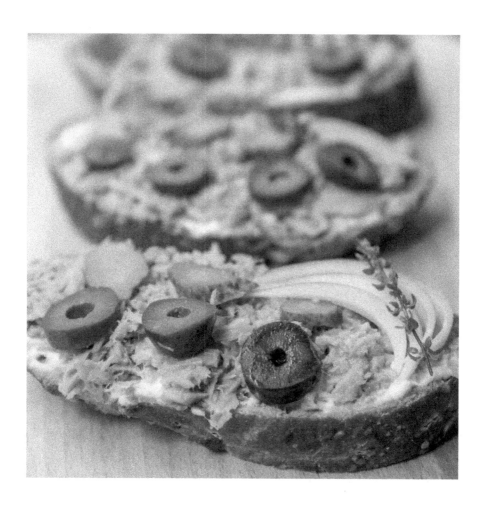

Open-Faced Margherita Sandwiches

Prep time: 10 minutes | Cook time: 5 minutes | Serves 4

Ingredients:
2 (6- to 7-inch) whole-wheat submarine or hoagie rolls, sliced open horizontally
1 tablespoon extra-virgin olive oil
1 garlic clove, halved
1 large ripe tomato, cut into 8 slices
¼ teaspoon dried oregano
1 cup fresh Mozzarella, sliced
¼ cup lightly packed fresh basil leaves, torn into small pieces
¼ teaspoon freshly ground black pepper

Directions:
Preheat the broiler to High with the rack 4 inches under the heating element.
Put the sliced bread on a large, rimmed baking sheet and broil for 1 minute, or until the bread is just lightly toasted. Remove from the oven. Brush each piece of the toasted bread with the oil, and rub a garlic half over each piece.
Put the toasted bread back on the baking sheet. Evenly divide the tomato slices on each piece. Sprinkle with the oregano and top with the cheese.
Place the baking sheet under the broiler. Set the timer for 1½ minutes, but check after 1 minute. When the cheese is melted and the edges are just starting to get dark brown, remove the sandwiches from the oven. Top each sandwich with the fresh basil and pepper before serving.

Per Serving:
calories: 93 | fat: 2.0g | protein: 10.0g | carbs: 8.0g | fiber: 2.0g | sodium: 313mg

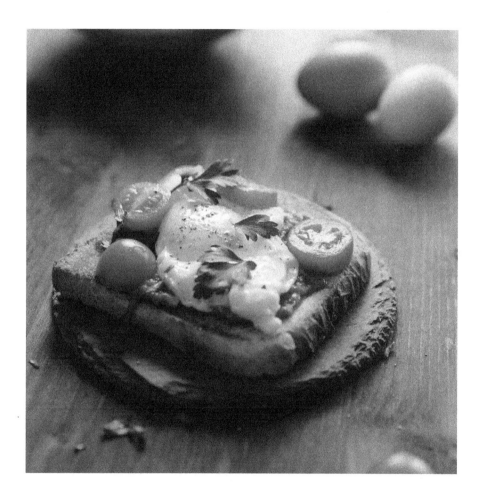

Grilled Caesar Salad Sandwiches

Prep time: 5 minutes | Cook time: 5 minutes | Serves 2

Ingredients:
¾ cup olive oil, divided
romaine lettuce hearts, left intact
to 4 anchovy fillets
Juice of 1 lemon
2 to 3 cloves garlic, peeled
teaspoon Dijon mustard
¼ teaspoon Worcestershire sauce
Sea salt and freshly ground pepper, to taste
slices whole-wheat bread, toasted
Freshly grated Parmesan cheese, for serving

Directions:
Preheat the grill to medium-high heat and oil the grates.
On a cutting board, drizzle the lettuce with 1 to 2 tablespoons of olive oil and place on the grates.
Grill for 5 minutes, turning until lettuce is slightly charred on all sides. Let lettuce cool enough to handle.
In a food processor, combine the remaining olive oil with the anchovies, lemon juice, garlic, mustard, and Worcestershire sauce.
Pulse the ingredients until you have a smooth emulsion. Season with sea salt and freshly ground pepper to taste. Chop the lettuce in half and place on the bread.
Drizzle with the dressing and serve with a sprinkle of Parmesan cheese.

Per Serving:
calories: 949 | fat: 85.6g | protein: 12.9g | carbs: 34.1g | fiber: 13.9g | sodium: 786mg

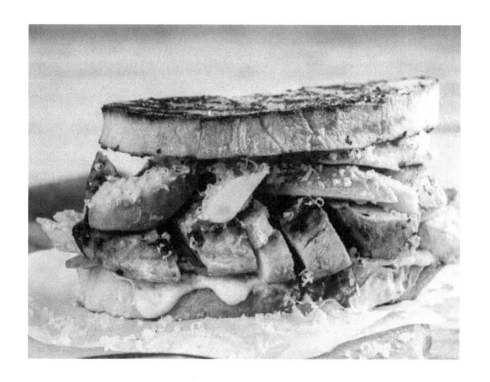

Green Veggie Sandwiches

Prep time: 20 minutes | Cook time: 0 minutes | Serves 2

Ingredients:

(15-ounce / 425-g) can cannellini beans, drained and rinsed

⅓ cup packed fresh basil leaves

⅓ cup packed fresh parsley

⅓ cup chopped fresh chives

garlic cloves, chopped

Zest and juice of ½ lemon

1 tablespoon apple cider vinegar Sandwiches:

4 whole-grain bread slices, toasted

8 English cucumber slices

1 large beefsteak tomato, cut into slices

1 large avocado, halved, pitted, and cut into slices

small yellow bell pepper, cut into slices

handfuls broccoli sprouts

2 handfuls fresh spinach

Directions:

In a food processor, combine the cannellini beans, basil, parsley, chives, garlic, lemon zest and juice, and vinegar. Pulse a few times, scrape down the sides, and purée until smooth. You may need to scrape down the sides again to incorporate all the basil and parsley. Refrigerate for at least 1 hour to allow the flavors to blend.

Assemble the Sandwiches Build your sandwiches by spreading several tablespoons of spread on each slice of bread. Layer two slices of bread with the cucumber, tomato, avocado, bell pepper, broccoli sprouts, and spinach. Top with the remaining bread slices and press down lightly. Serve immediately.

Per Serving: calories: 617 | fat: 21.1g | protein: 28.1g | carbs: 86.1g | fiber: 25.6g | sodium: 593mg

Beans, Grains, and Pastas

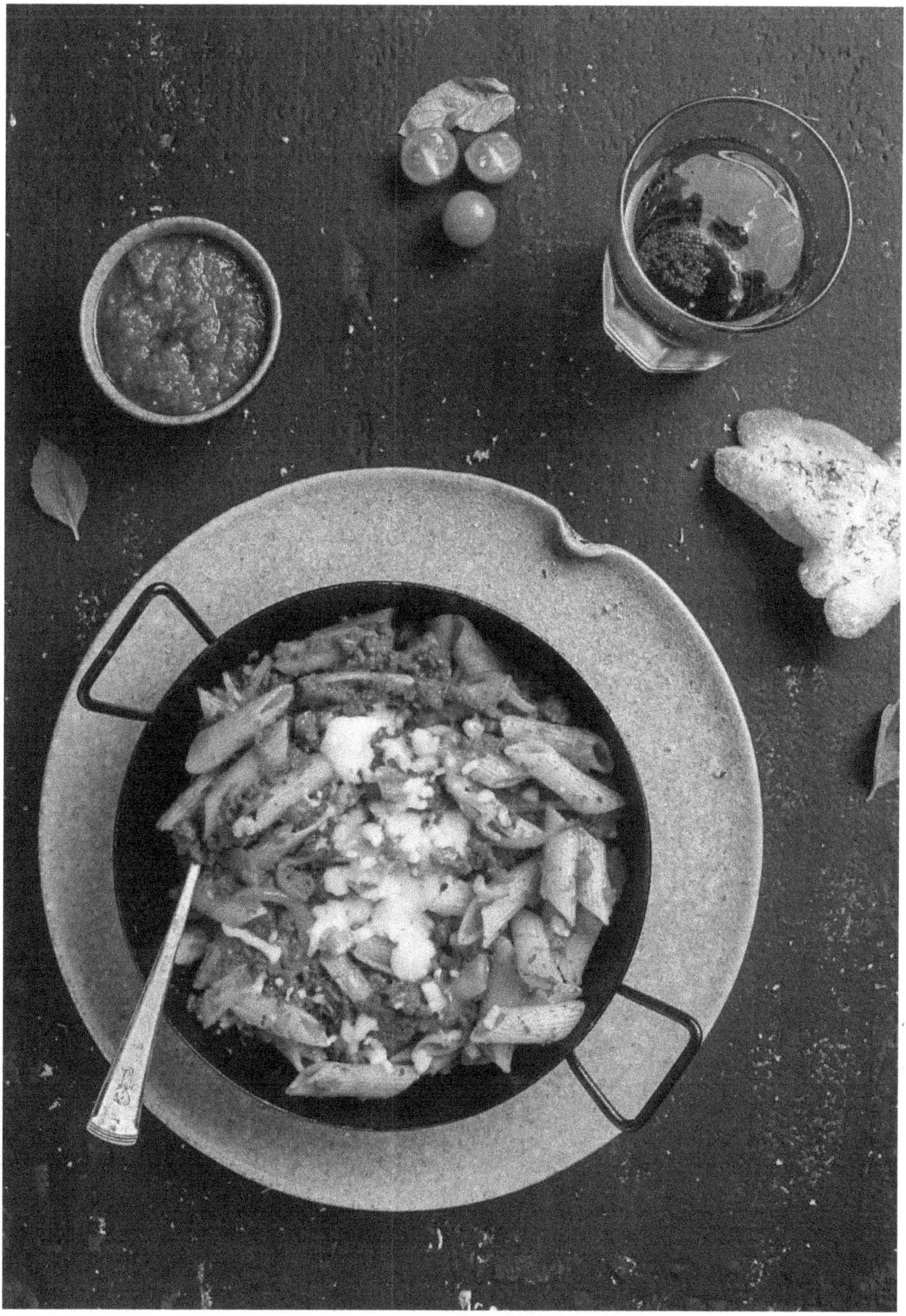

Black Bean Chili with Mangoes

Prep time: 10 minutes | Cook time: 10 minutes | Serves 4

Ingredients:
2 tablespoons coconut oil
onion, chopped
(15-ounce / 425-g) cans black beans, drained and rinsed
1 tablespoon chili powder
1 teaspoon sea salt
¼ teaspoon freshly ground black pepper
cup water
ripe mangoes, sliced thinly
¼ cup chopped fresh cilantro, divided
¼ cup sliced scallions, divided

Directions:
Heat the coconut oil in a pot over high heat until melted.
Put the onion in the pot and sauté for 5 minutes or until translucent.
Add the black beans to the pot. Sprinkle with chili powder, salt, and
ground black pepper. Pour in the water. Stir to mix well.
Bring to a boil. Reduce the heat to low, then simmering for 5 minutes
or until the beans are tender.
Turn off the heat and mix in the mangoes, then garnish with scallions
and cilantro before serving.

Per Serving:
calories: 430 | fat: 9.1g | protein: 20.2g | carbs: 71.9g | fiber: 22.0g |
sodium: 608mg

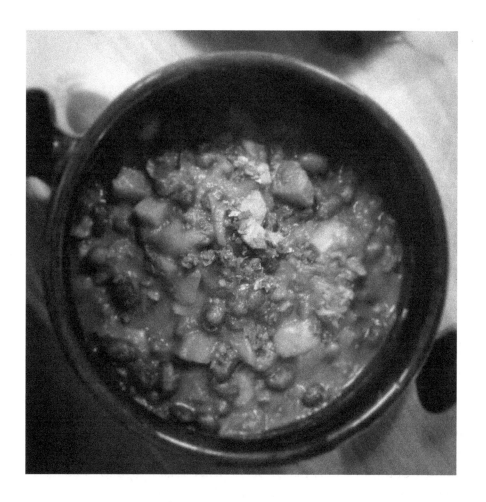

Slow Cooked Turkey and Brown Rice

Prep time: 20 minutes | Cook time: 3 hours 10 minutes | Serves 6

Ingredients:
tablespoon extra-virgin olive oil
1½ pounds (680 g) ground turkey
tablespoons chopped fresh sage, divided
2 tablespoons chopped fresh thyme, divided
teaspoon sea salt
½ teaspoon ground black pepper
cups brown rice
1 (14-ounce / 397-g) can stewed tomatoes, with the juice
¼ cup pitted and sliced Kalamata olives
3 medium zucchini, sliced thinly
¼ cup chopped fresh flat-leaf parsley
1 medium yellow onion, chopped
tablespoon plus 1 teaspoon balsamic vinegar
cups low-sodium chicken stock
2 garlic cloves, minced
½ cup grated Parmesan cheese, for serving

Directions:
Heat the olive oil in a nonstick skillet over medium-high heat until shimmering. Add the ground turkey and sprinkle with 1 tablespoon of sage, 1 tablespoon of thyme, salt and ground black pepper. Sauté for 10 minutes or until the ground turkey is lightly browned. Pour them in the slow cooker, then pour in the remaining ingredients, except for the Parmesan. Stir to mix well. Put the lid on and cook on high for 3 hours or until the rice and vegetables are tender. Pour them in a large serving bowl, then spread with Parmesan cheese before serving.

Per Serving:
calories: 499 | fat: 16.4g | protein: 32.4g | carbs: 56.5g | fiber: 4.7g | sodium: 758mg

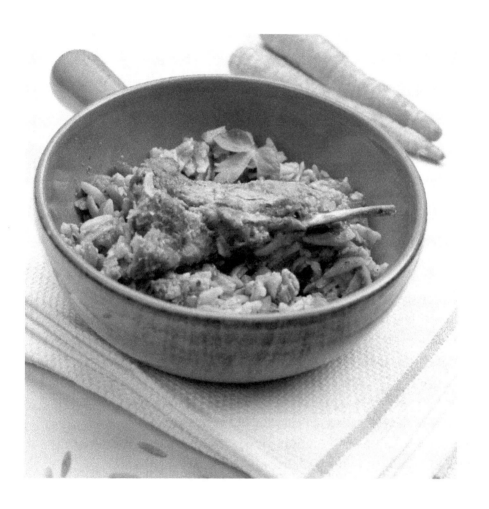

Papaya, Jicama, and Peas Rice Bowl
Prep time: 20 minutes | Cook time: 45 minutes | Serves 4

Sauce:
Juice of ¼ lemon
2 teaspoons chopped fresh basil
1 tablespoon raw honey
tablespoon extra-virgin olive oil
Sea salt, to taste

Rice:
1½ cups wild rice
papayas, peeled, seeded, and diced
1 jicama, peeled and shredded
cup snow peas, julienned
cups shredded cabbage
1 scallion, white and green parts, chopped

Directions:
Combine the ingredients for the sauce in a bowl. Stir to mix well. Set aside until ready to use.
Pour the wild rice in a saucepan, then pour in enough water to cover. Bring to a boil.
Reduce the heat to low, then simmer for 45 minutes or until the wild rice is soft and plump. Drain and transfer to a large serving bowl.
Top the rice with papayas, jicama, peas, cabbage, and scallion. Pour the sauce over and stir to mix well before serving.

Per Serving:
calories: 446 | fat: 7.9g | protein: 13.1g | carbs: 85.8g | fiber: 16.0g | sodium: 70mg

---

Garlic Shrimp Fettuccine

Prep time: 10 minutes | Cook time: 15 minutes | Serves 4 to 6

Ingredients:
8 ounces (227 g) fettuccine pasta
¼ cup extra-virgin olive oil
3 tablespoons garlic, minced
1 pound (454 g) large shrimp, peeled and deveined
⅓ cup lemon juice
1 tablespoon lemon zest
½ teaspoon salt
½ teaspoon freshly ground black pepper

Directions:
Bring a large pot of salted water to a boil. Add the fettuccine and cook for 8 minutes. Reserve ½ cup of the cooking liquid and drain the pasta. In a large saucepan over medium heat, heat the olive oil. Add the garlic and sauté for 1 minute.
Add the shrimp to the saucepan and cook each side for 3 minutes. Remove the shrimp from the pan and set aside.
Add the remaining ingredients to the saucepan. Stir in the cooking liquid. Add the pasta and toss together to evenly coat the pasta. Transfer the pasta to a serving dish and serve topped with the cooked shrimp.

Per Serving:
calories: 615 | fat: 17.0g | protein: 33.0g | carbs: 89.0g | fiber: 4.0g | sodium: 407mg

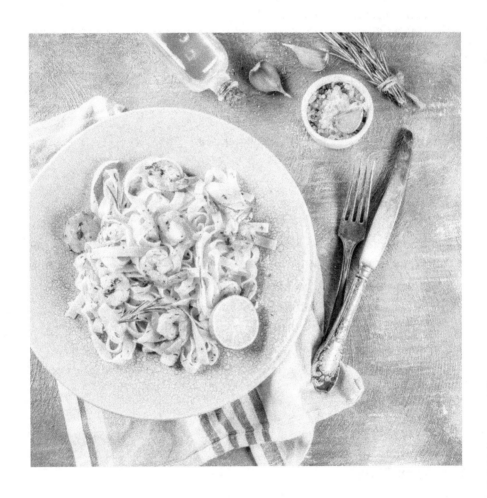

Pesto Pasta

Prep time: 10 minutes | Cook time: 8 minutes | Serves 4 to 6

Ingredients:

1 pound (454 g) spaghetti
4 cups fresh basil leaves, stems removed
3 cloves garlic
1 teaspoon salt
½ teaspoon freshly ground black pepper
½ cup toasted pine nuts
¼ cup lemon juice
½ cup grated Parmesan cheese
1 cup extra-virgin olive oil

Directions:

Bring a large pot of salted water to a boil. Add the spaghetti to the pot and cook for 8 minutes.

In a food processor, place the remaining ingredients, except for the olive oil, and pulse.

While the processor is running, slowly drizzle the olive oil through the top opening. Process until all the olive oil has been added.

Reserve ½ cup of the cooking liquid. Drain the pasta and put it into a large bowl. Add the pesto and cooking liquid to the bowl of pasta and toss everything together.

Serve immediately.

Per Serving:

calories: 1067 | fat: 72.0g | protein: 23.0g | carbs: 91..0g | fiber: 6.0g | sodium: 817mg

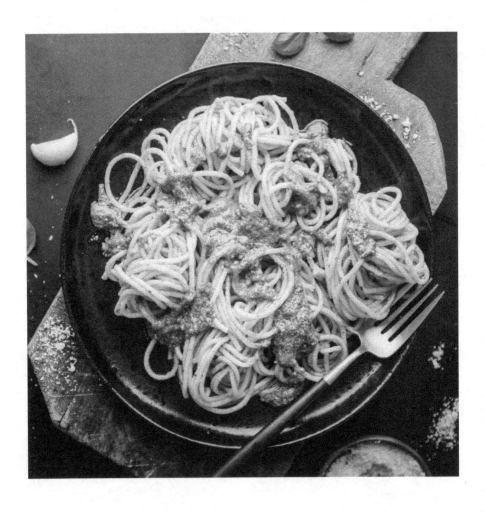

Cumin Quinoa Pilaf

Prep time: 5 minutes | Cook time: 5 minutes | Serves 2

Ingredients:
2 tablespoons extra virgin olive oil
cloves garlic, minced
cups water
2 cups quinoa, rinsed
2 teaspoons ground cumin
2 teaspoons turmeric
Salt, to taste
1 handful parsley, chopped

Directions:
Press the Sauté button to heat your Instant Pot.
Once hot, add the oil and garlic to the pot, stir and cook for 1 minute.
Add water, quinoa, cumin, turmeric, and salt, stirring well.
Lock the lid. Select the Manual mode and set the cooking time for 1
minute at High Pressure.
When the timer beeps, perform a natural pressure release for 10
minutes, then release any remaining pressure. Carefully remove the lid.
Fluff the quinoa with a fork. Season with more salt, if needed.
Sprinkle the chopped parsley on top and serve.

Per Serving:
calories: 384 | fat: 12.3g | protein: 12.8g | carbs: 57.4g | fiber: 6.9g |
sodium: 448mg

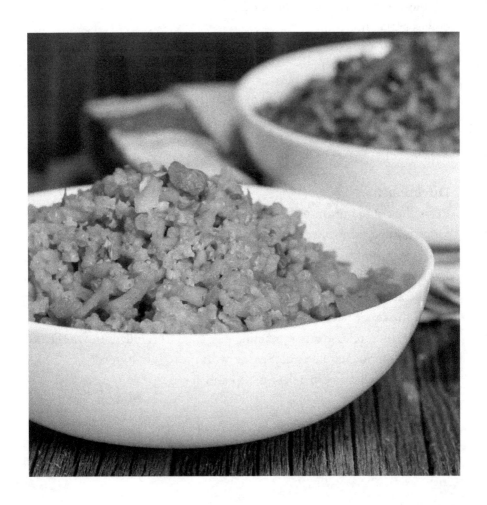

Vegetable Mains

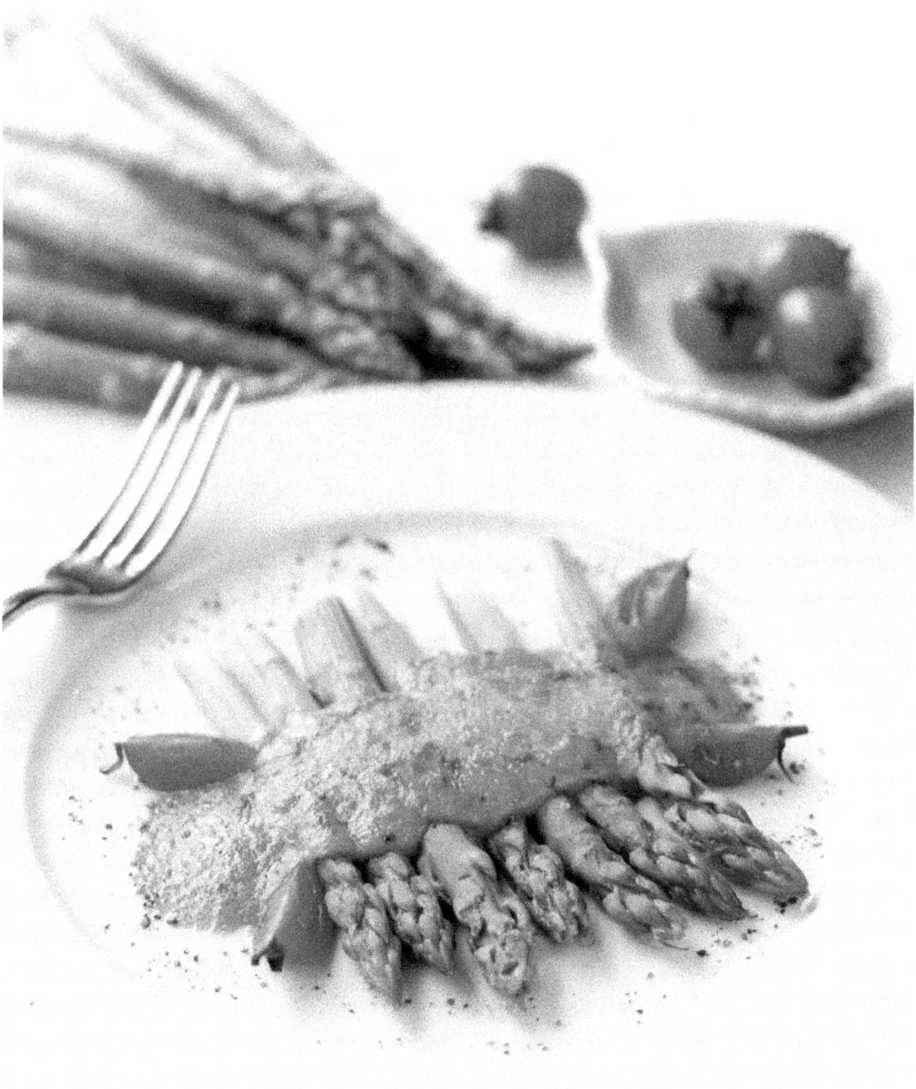

Cauliflower Hash with Carrots

Prep time: 10 minutes | Cook time: 10 minutes | Serves 4

Ingredients:

3 tablespoons extra-virgin olive oil
1 large onion, chopped
tablespoon minced garlic
cups diced carrots
4 cups cauliflower florets
½ teaspoon ground cumin
1 teaspoon salt

Directions:

In a large skillet, heat the olive oil over medium heat.
Add the onion and garlic and saut é for 1 minute. Stir in the carrots and stir-fry for 3 minutes.
Add the cauliflower florets, cumin, and salt and toss to combine.
Cover and cook for 3 minutes until lightly browned. Stir well and cook, uncovered, for 3 to 4 minutes, until softened.
Remove from the heat and serve warm.

Per Serving:

calories: 158 | fat: 10.8g | protein: 3.1g | carbs: 14.9g | fiber: 5.1g | sodium: 656mg

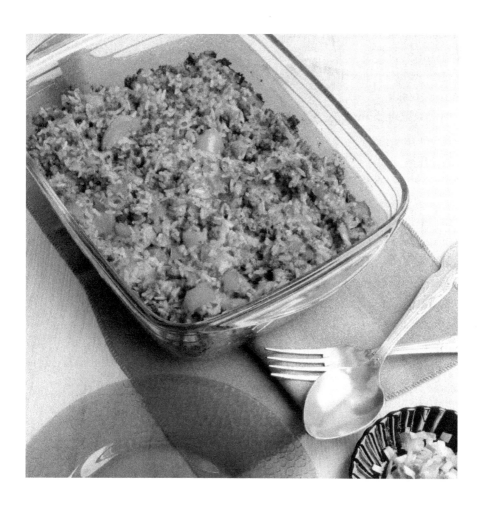

Garlicky Zucchini Cubes with Mint

Prep time: 5 minutes | Cook time: 10 minutes | Serves 4

Ingredients:
3 large green zucchini, cut into ½-inch cubes
3 tablespoons extra-virgin olive oil
1 large onion, chopped
3 cloves garlic, minced
1 teaspoon salt
1 teaspoon dried mint

Directions:
Heat the olive oil in a large skillet over medium heat.
Add the onion and garlic and saut é for 3 minutes, stirring constantly, or until softened.
Stir in the zucchini cubes and salt and cook for 5 minutes, or until the zucchini is browned and tender.
Add the mint to the skillet and toss to combine, then continue cooking for 2 minutes.
Serve warm.

Per Serving:
calories: 146 | fat: 10.6g | protein: 4.2g | carbs: 11.8g | fiber: 3.0g | sodium: 606mg

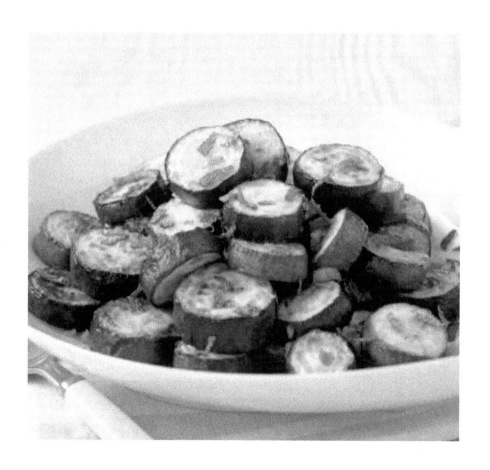

Stuffed Portobello Mushrooms with Spinach

Prep time: 5 minutes | Cook time: 20 minutes | Serves 4

Ingredients:
8 large portobello mushrooms, stems removed
3 teaspoons extra-virgin olive oil, divided
1 medium red bell pepper, diced
4 cups fresh spinach
¼ cup crumbled feta cheese

Directions:
Preheat the oven to 450°F (235°C).
Using a spoon to scoop out the gills of the mushrooms and discard them. Brush the mushrooms with 2 teaspoons of olive oil.
Arrange the mushrooms (cap-side down) on a baking sheet. Roast in the preheated oven for 20 minutes.
Meantime, in a medium skillet, heat the remaining olive oil over medium heat until it shimmers.
Add the bell pepper and spinach and saut é for 8 to 10 minutes, stirring occasionally, or until the spinach is wilted.
Remove the mushrooms from the oven to a paper towel-lined plate. Using a spoon to stuff each mushroom with the bell pepper and spinach mixture. Scatter the feta cheese all over.
Serve immediately.

Per Serving:
calories: 115 | fat: 5.9g | protein: 7.2g | carbs: 11.5g | fiber: 4.0g | sodium: 125mg

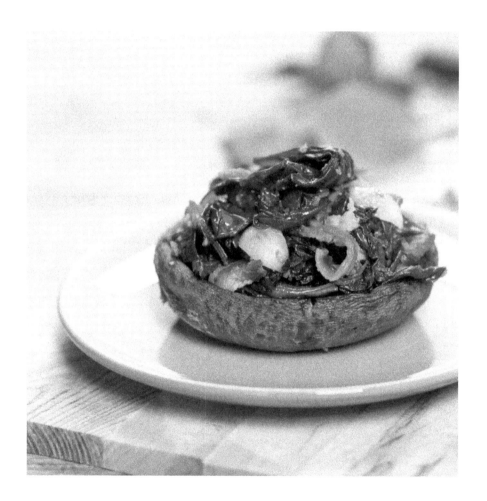

Chickpea Lettuce Wraps with Celery

Prep time: 10 minutes | Cook time: 0 minutes | Serves 4

Ingredients:
1 (15-ounce / 425-g) can low-sodium chickpeas, drained and rinsed
celery stalk, thinly sliced
tablespoons finely chopped red onion
tablespoons unsalted tahini
tablespoons honey mustard
1 tablespoon capers, undrained
12 butter lettuce leaves

Directions:
In a bowl, mash the chickpeas with a potato masher or the back of a fork until mostly smooth.
Add the celery, red onion, tahini, honey mustard, and capers to the bowl and stir until well incorporated.
For each serving, place three overlapping lettuce leaves on a plate and top with ¼ of the mashed chickpea filling, then roll up. Repeat with the remaining lettuce leaves and chickpea mixture.

Per Serving:
calories: 182 | fat: 7.1g | protein: 10.3g | carbs: 19.6g | fiber: 3.0g | sodium: 171mg

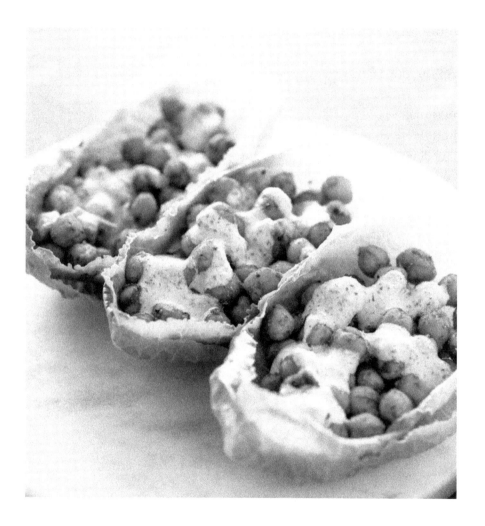

Parmesan Stuffed Zucchini Boats

Prep time: 5 minutes | Cook time: 15 minutes | Serves 4

Ingredients:
1 cup canned low-sodium chickpeas, drained and rinsed
cup no-sugar-added spaghetti sauce
zucchinis
¼ cup shredded Parmesan cheese

Directions:
Preheat the oven to 425°F (220°C).
In a medium bowl, stir together the chickpeas and spaghetti sauce.
Cut the zucchini in half lengthwise and scrape a spoon gently down the length of each half to remove the seeds.
Fill each zucchini half with the chickpea sauce and top with one-quarter of the Parmesan cheese.
Place the zucchini halves on a baking sheet and roast in the oven for 15 minutes.
Transfer to a plate. Let rest for 5 minutes before serving.

Per Serving:
calories: 139 | fat: 4.0g | protein: 8.0g | carbs: 20.0g | fiber: 5.0g | sodium: 344mg

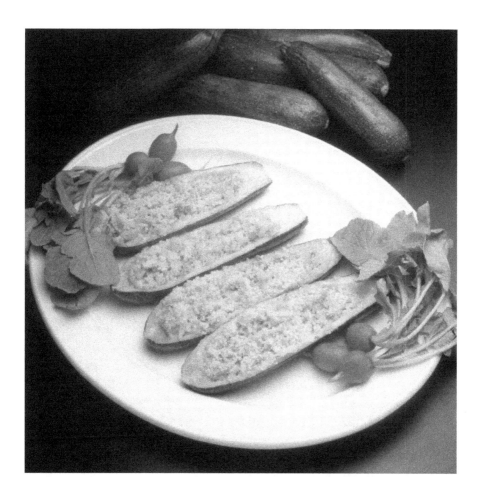

Baby Kale and Cabbage Salad

Prep time: 10 minutes | Cook time: 0 minutes | Serves 6

Ingredients:
2 bunches baby kale, thinly sliced
½ head green savoy cabbage, cored and thinly sliced
1 medium red bell pepper, thinly sliced
1 garlic clove, thinly sliced
1 cup toasted peanuts Dressing:
Juice of 1 lemon
¼ cup apple cider vinegar
1 teaspoon ground cumin
¼ teaspoon smoked paprika

Directions:
In a large mixing bowl, toss together the kale and cabbage.
Make the dressing: Whisk together the lemon juice, vinegar, cumin and paprika in a small bowl.
Pour the dressing over the greens and gently massage with your hands.
Add the pepper, garlic and peanuts to the mixing bowl. Toss to combine.
Serve immediately.

Per Serving:
calories: 199 | fat: 12.0g | protein: 10.0g | carbs: 17.0g | fiber: 5.0g | sodium: 46mg

Poultry and Meats

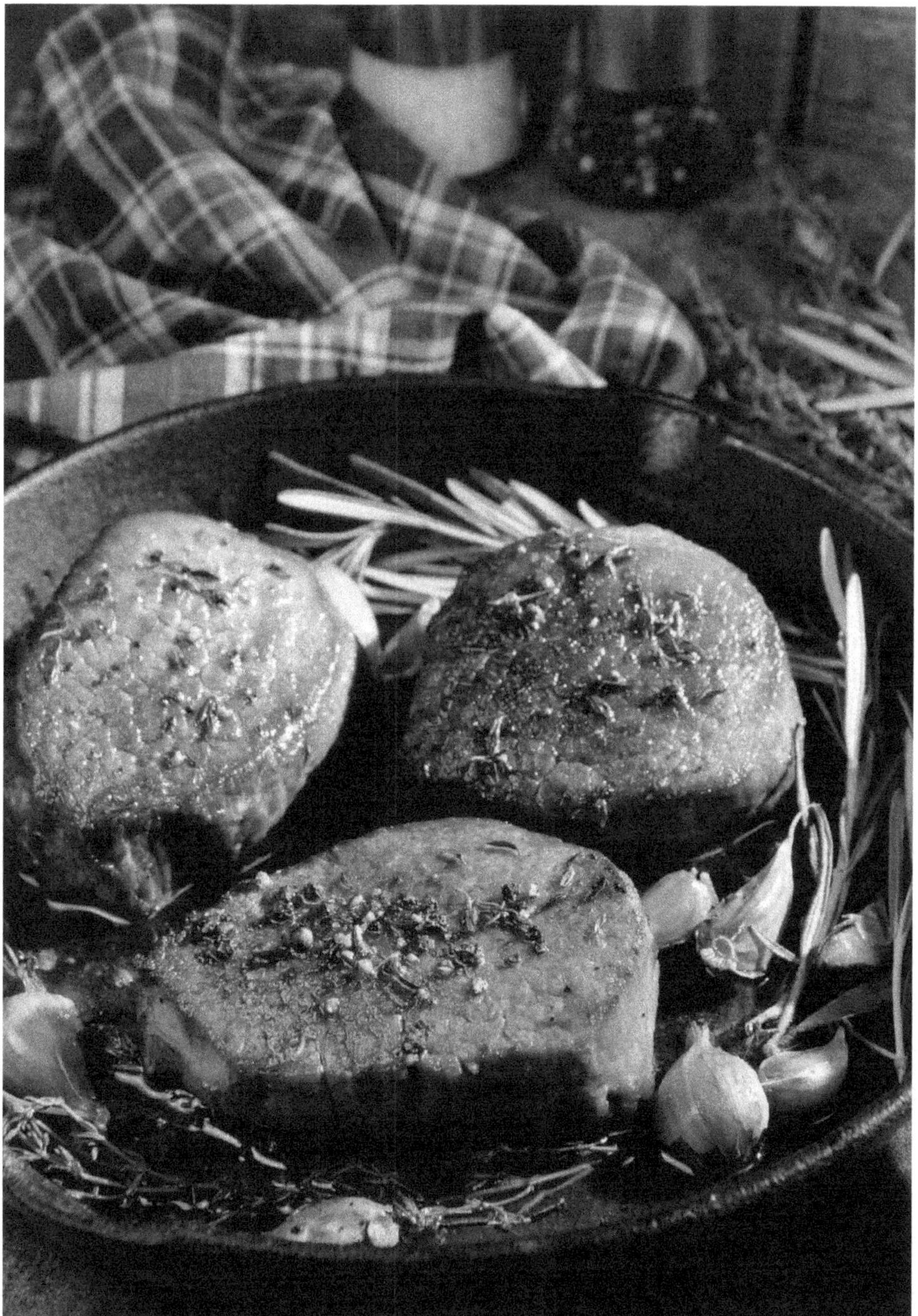

Spiced Roast Chicken

Prep time: 10 minutes | Cook time: 35 minutes | Serves 6

Ingredients:
1 teaspoon garlic powder
1 teaspoon ground paprika
½ teaspoon ground cumin
½ teaspoon ground coriander
½ teaspoon salt
¼ teaspoon ground cayenne pepper
6 chicken legs
1 teaspoon extra-virgin olive oil

Directions:
Preheat the oven to 400°F (205°C).
Combine the garlic powder, paprika, cumin, coriander, salt, and cayenne pepper in a small bowl.
On a clean work surface, rub the spices all over the chicken legs until completely coated.
Heat the olive oil in an ovenproof skillet over medium heat.
Add the chicken thighs and sear each side for 8 to 10 minutes, or until the skin is crispy and browned.
Transfer the skillet to the preheated oven and continue cooking for 10 to 15 minutes, or until the juices run clear and it registers an internal temperature of 165°F (74°C).
Remove from the heat and serve on plates.

Per Serving:
calories: 275 | fat: 15.6g | protein: 30.3g | carbs: 0.9g | fiber: 0g | sodium: 255mg

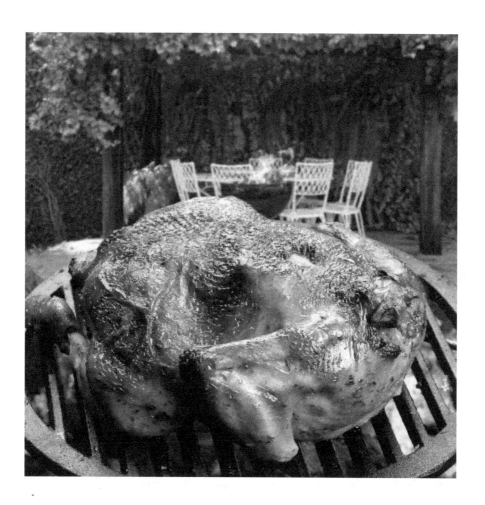

Yogurt Chicken Breasts

Prep time: 10 minutes | Cook time: 10 minutes | Serves 4

Ingredients:
1 pound (454 g) boneless, skinless chicken breasts, cut into 2-inch strips
tablespoon extra-virgin olive oil
Yogurt Sauce:
½ cup plain Greek yogurt
tablespoons water
Pinch saffron (3 or 4 threads)
garlic cloves, minced
½ onion, chopped
2 tablespoons chopped fresh cilantro
Juice of ½ lemon
½ teaspoon salt

Directions:
Make the yogurt sauce: Place the yogurt, water, saffron, garlic, onion, cilantro, lemon juice, and salt in a blender, and pulse until completely mixed.
Transfer the yogurt sauce to a large bowl, along with the chicken strips. Toss to coat well.
Cover with plastic wrap and marinate in the refrigerator for at least 1 hour, or up to overnight.
When ready to cook, heat the olive oil in a large skillet over medium heat.
Add the chicken strips to the skillet, discarding any excess marinade. Cook each side for 5 minutes, or until cooked through.
Let the chicken cool for 5 minutes before serving.

Per Serving:
calories: 154 | fat: 4.8g | protein: 26.3g | carbs: 2.9g | fiber: 0g | sodium: 500mg

Greek-Style Lamb Burgers

Prep time: 10 minutes | Cook time: 10 minutes | Serves 4

Ingredients:
1 pound (454 g) ground lamb
½ teaspoon salt
½ teaspoon freshly ground black pepper
4 tablespoons crumbled feta cheese
Buns, toppings, and tzatziki, for serving (optional)

Directions:
Preheat the grill to high heat.
In a large bowl, using your hands, combine the lamb with the salt and pepper.
Divide the meat into 4 portions. Divide each portion in half to make a top and a bottom. Flatten each half into a 3-inch circle. Make a dent in the center of one of the halves and place 1 tablespoon of the feta cheese in the center. Place the second half of the patty on top of the feta cheese and press down to close the 2 halves together, making it resemble a round burger.
Grill each side for 3 minutes, for medium-well. Serve on a bun with your favorite toppings and tzatziki sauce, if desired.

Per Serving:
calories: 345 | fat: 29.0g | protein: 20.0g | carbs: 1.0g | fiber: 0g | sodium: 462mg

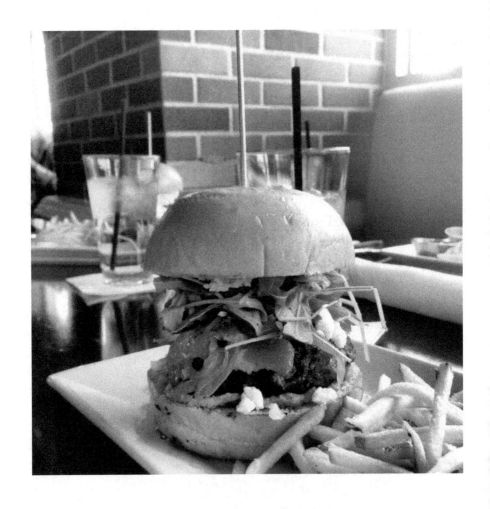

Chicken Bruschetta Burgers

Prep time: 10 minutes | Cook time: 16 minutes | Serves 2

Ingredients:
tablespoon olive oil
garlic cloves, minced
tablespoons finely minced onion
1 teaspoon dried basil
3 tablespoons minced sun-dried tomatoes packed in olive oil
8 ounces (227 g) ground chicken breast
¼ teaspoon salt
3 pieces small Mozzarella balls, minced

Directions:
Heat the olive oil in a nonstick skillet over medium-high heat. Add the garlic and onion and sauté for 5 minutes until tender. Stir in the basil. Remove from the skillet to a medium bowl.
Add the tomatoes, ground chicken, and salt and stir until incorporated. Mix in the Mozzarella balls.
Divide the chicken mixture in half and form into two burgers, each about ¾-inch thick.
Heat the same skillet over medium-high heat and add the burgers. Cook each side for 5 to 6 minutes, or until they reach an internal temperature of 165°F (74°C).
Serve warm.

Per Serving:
calories: 300 | fat: 17.0g | protein: 32.2g | carbs: 6.0g | fiber: 1.1g | sodium: 724mg

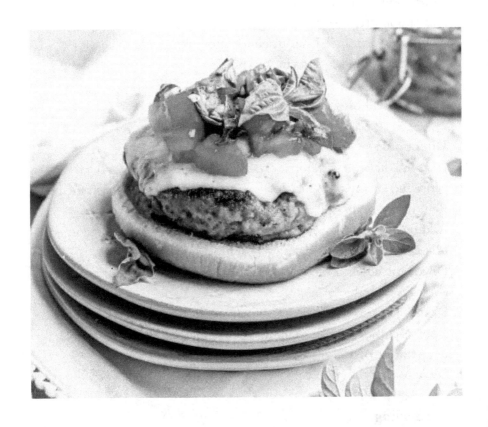

Herbed-Mustard-Coated Pork Tenderloin

Prep time: 10 minutes | Cook time: 15 minutes | Serves 4

Ingredients:
3 tablespoons fresh rosemary leaves
¼ cup Dijon mustard
½ cup fresh parsley leaves
6 garlic cloves
½ teaspoon sea salt
¼ teaspoon freshly ground black pepper
1 tablespoon extra-virgin olive oil
1 (1½-pound / 680-g) pork tenderloin

Directions:
Preheat the oven to 400°F (205°C).

Put all the ingredients, except for the pork tenderloin, in a food processor. Pulse until it has a thick consistency.

Put the pork tenderloin on a baking sheet, then rub with the mixture to coat well.

Put the sheet in the preheated oven and bake for 15 minutes or until the internal temperature of the pork reaches at least 165°F (74°C). Flip the tenderloin halfway through the cooking time.

Transfer the cooked pork tenderloin to a large plate and allow to cool for 5 minutes before serving.

Per Serving:
calories: 363 | fat: 18.1g | protein: 2.2g | carbs: 4.9g | fiber: 2.0g | sodium: 514mg

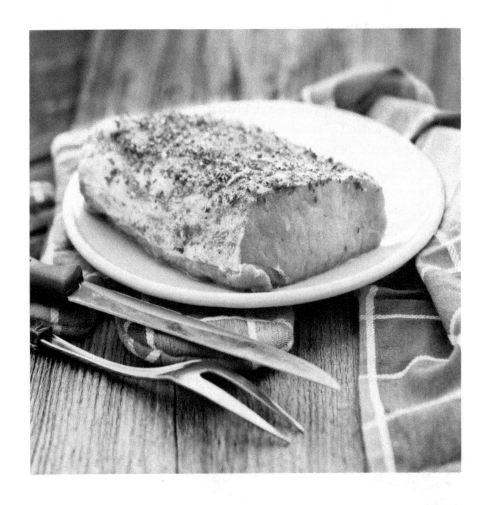

Fish and Seafood

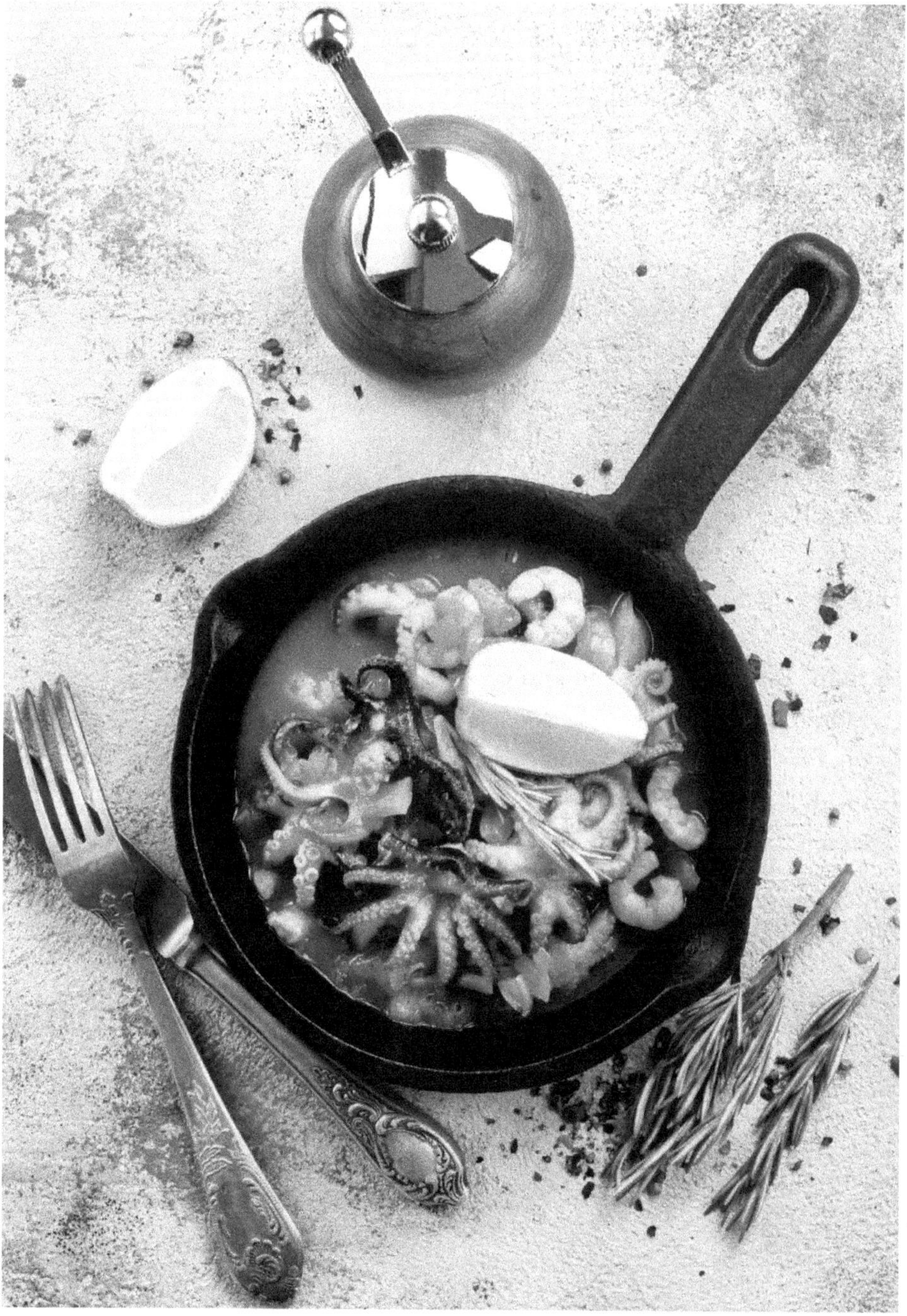

Mediterranean Braised Cod with Vegetables

Prep time: 10 minutes | Cook time: 18 minutes | Serves 2

Ingredients:
tablespoon olive oil
½ medium onion, minced
garlic cloves, minced
1 teaspoon oregano
1 (15-ounce / 425-g) can artichoke hearts in water, drained and halved
1 (15-ounce / 425-g) can diced tomatoes with basil
¼ cup pitted Greek olives, drained
10 ounces (284 g) wild cod
Salt and freshly ground black pepper, to taste

Directions:
In a skillet, heat the olive oil over medium-high heat.
Saut é the onion for about 5 minutes, stirring occasionally, or until tender.
Stir in the garlic and oregano and cook for 30 seconds more until fragrant.
Add the artichoke hearts, tomatoes, and olives and stir to combine.
Top with the cod.
Cover and cook for 10 minutes, or until the fish flakes easily with a fork and juices run clean.
Sprinkle with the salt and pepper. Serve warm.

Per Serving:
calories: 332 | fat: 10.5g | protein: 29.2g | carbs: 30.7g | fiber: 8.0g | sodium: 1906mg

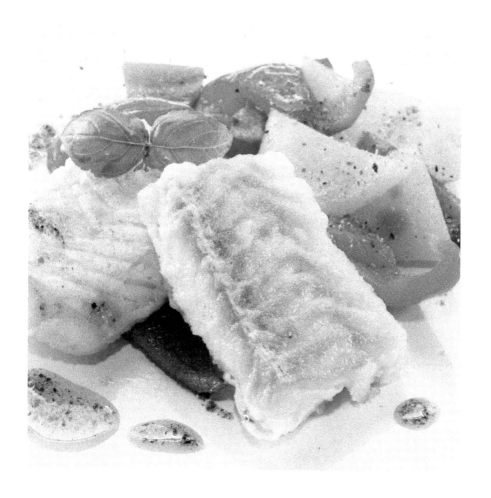

Lemon-Parsley Swordfish

Prep time: 10 minutes | Cook time: 17 to 20 minutes | Serves 4

Ingredients:
cup fresh Italian parsley
¼ cup lemon juice
¼ cup extra-virgin olive oil
¼ cup fresh thyme
cloves garlic
½ teaspoon salt
4 swordfish steaks
Olive oil spray

Directions:
Preheat the oven to 450°F (235°C). Grease a large baking dish generously with olive oil spray.
Place the parsley, lemon juice, olive oil, thyme, garlic, and salt in a food processor and pulse until smoothly blended.
Arrange the swordfish steaks in the greased baking dish and spoon the parsley mixture over the top.
Bake in the preheated oven for 17 to 20 minutes until flaky.
Divide the fish among four plates and serve hot.

Per Serving:
calories: 396 | fat: 21.7g | protein: 44.2g | carbs: 2.9g | fiber: 1.0g | sodium: 494mg

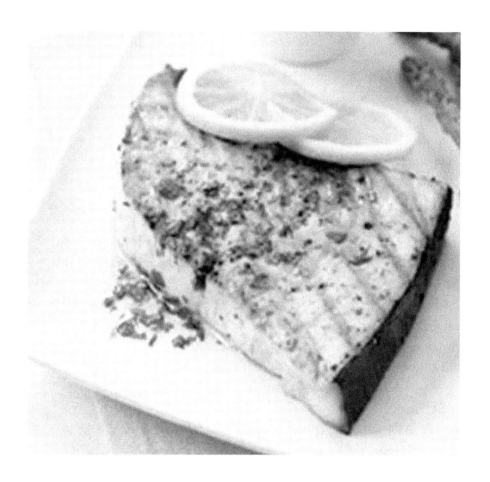

Spicy Grilled Shrimp with Lemon Wedges

Prep time: 15 minutes | Cook time: 6 minutes | Serves 6

Ingredients:
1 large clove garlic, crushed
1 teaspoon coarse salt
teaspoon paprika
½ teaspoon cayenne pepper
teaspoons lemon juice
2 tablespoons plus 1 teaspoon olive oil, divided
2 pounds (907 g) large shrimp, peeled and deveined
8 wedges lemon, for garnish

Directions:
Preheat the grill to medium heat.
Stir together the garlic, salt, paprika, cayenne pepper, lemon juice, and 2 tablespoons of olive oil in a small bowl until a paste forms. Add the shrimp and toss until well coated.
Grease the grill grates lightly with remaining 1 teaspoon of olive oil. Grill the shrimp for 4 to 6 minutes, flipping the shrimp halfway through, or until the shrimp is totally pink and opaque.
Garnish the shrimp with lemon wedges and serve hot.

Per Serving:
calories: 163 | fat: 5.8g | protein: 25.2g | carbs: 2.8g | fiber: 0.4g | sodium: 585mg

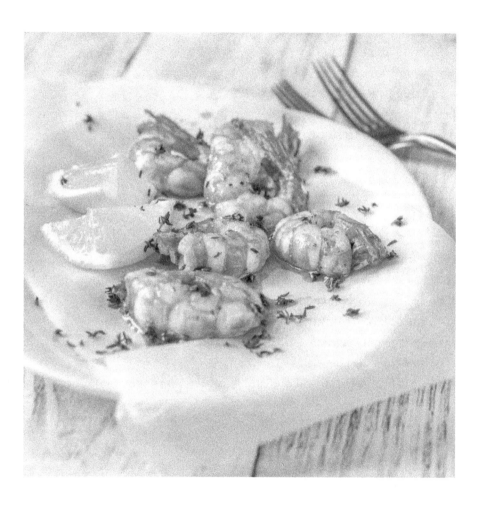

Orange Flavored Scallops

Prep time: 10 minutes | Cook time: 10 minutes | Serves 4

Ingredients:

2 pounds (907 g) sea scallops, patted dry

Sea salt and freshly ground black pepper, to taste

2 tablespoons extra-virgin olive oil

1 tablespoon minced garlic

¼ cup freshly squeezed orange juice

teaspoon orange zest

teaspoons chopped fresh thyme, for garnish

Directions:

In a bowl, lightly season the scallops with salt and pepper. Set aside.

Heat the olive oil in a large skillet over medium-high heat until it shimmers.

Add the garlic and saut é for about 3 minutes, or until fragrant.

Stir in the seasoned scallops and sear each side for about 4 minutes, or until the scallops are browned.

Remove the scallops from the heat to a plate and set aside.

Add the orange juice and zest to the skillet, scraping up brown bits from bottom of skillet.

Drizzle the sauce over the scallops and garnish with the thyme before serving.

Per Serving:

calories: 266 | fat: 7.6g | protein: 38.1g | carbs: 7.9g | fiber: 0g | sodium: 360mg

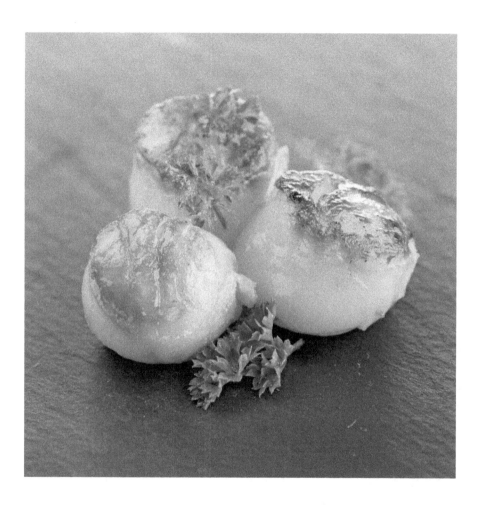

Haddock with Cucumber Sauce

Prep time: 10 minutes | Cook time: 10 minutes | Serves 4

Ingredients:
¼ cup plain Greek yogurt
½ scallion, white and green parts, finely chopped
½ English cucumber, grated, liquid squeezed out
2 teaspoons chopped fresh mint
1 teaspoon honey
Sea salt and freshly ground black pepper, to taste
4 (5-ounce / 142-g) haddock fillets, patted dry
Nonstick cooking spray

Directions:
In a small bowl, stir together the yogurt, cucumber, scallion, mint, honey, and a pinch of salt. Set aside.
Season the fillets lightly with salt and pepper.
Place a large skillet over medium-high heat and spray lightly with cooking spray.
Cook the haddock, turning once, until it is just cooked through, about 5 minutes per side.
Remove the fish from the heat and transfer to plates.
Serve topped with the cucumber sauce.

Per Serving:
calories: 164 | fat: 2.0g | protein: 27.0g | carbs: 4.0g | fiber: 0g | sodium: 104mg

Fruits and Desserts

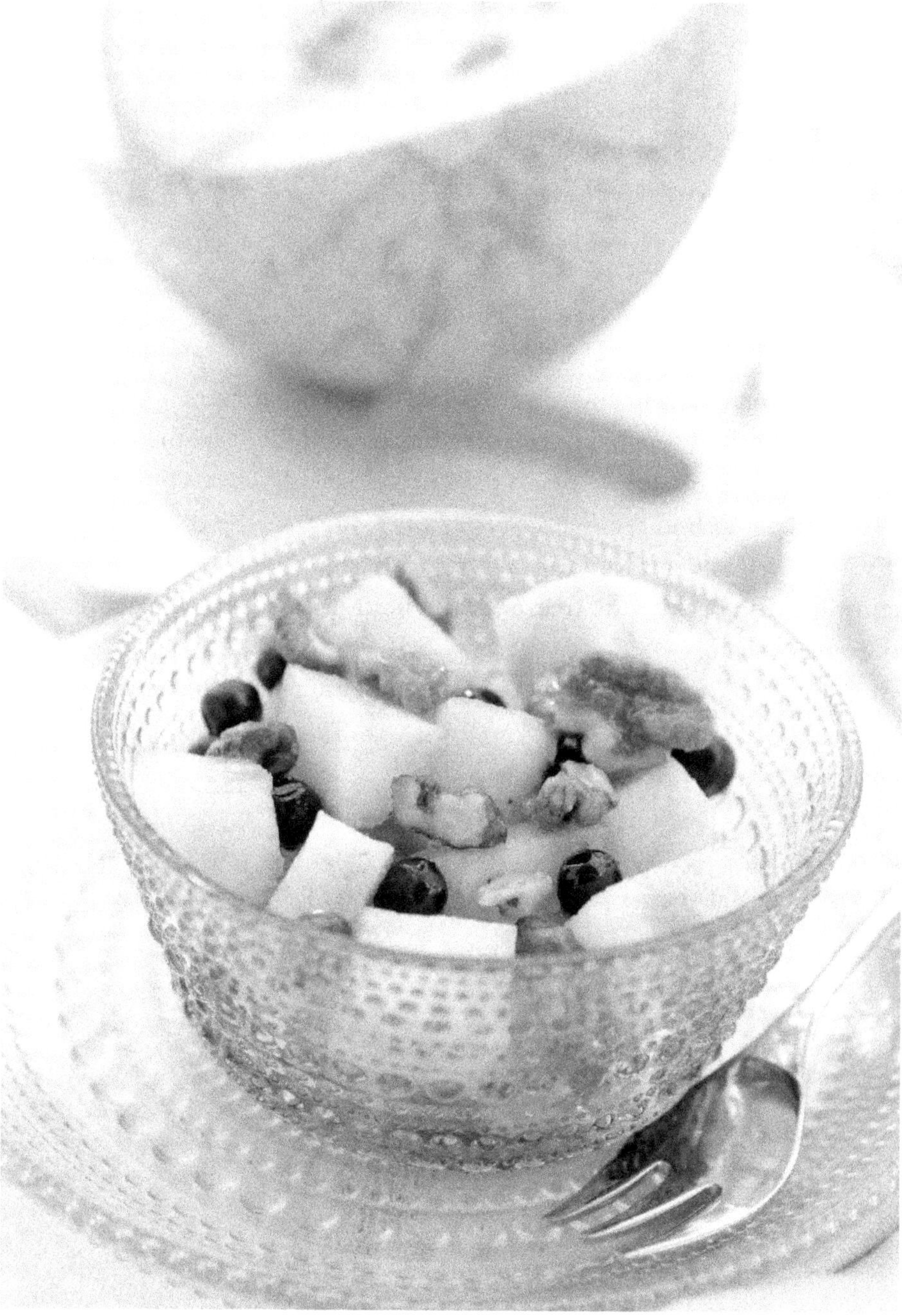

Lemony Blackberry Granita

Prep time: 10 minutes | Cook time: 0 minutes | Serves 4

Ingredients:
1 pound (454 g) fresh blackberries
1 teaspoon chopped fresh thyme
¼ cup freshly squeezed lemon juice
½ cup raw honey
½ cup water

Directions:
Put all the ingredients in a food processor, then pulse to purée.
Pour the mixture through a sieve into a baking dish. Discard the seeds remain in the sieve.
Put the baking dish in the freezer for 2 hours. Remove the dish from the refrigerator and stir to break any frozen parts.
Return the dish back to the freezer for an hour, then stir to break any frozen parts again.
Return the dish to the freezer for 4 hours until the granita is completely frozen.
Remove it from the freezer and mash to serve.

Per Serving:
calories: 183 | fat: 1.1g | protein: 2.2g | carbs: 45.9g | fiber: 6.0g | sodium: 6mg

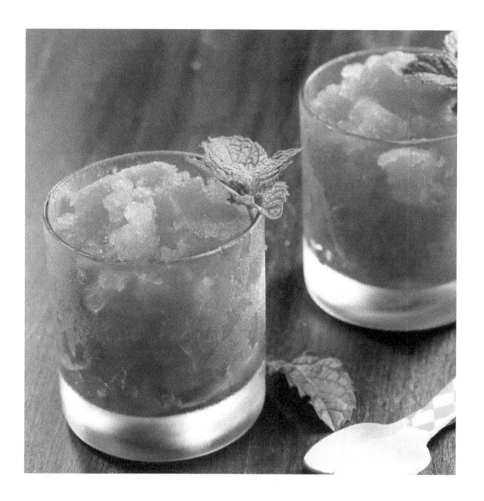

Lemony Tea and Chia Pudding

Prep time: 30 minutes | Cook time: 0 minutes | Serves 3 to 4

Ingredients:
2 teaspoons matcha green tea powder (optional)
2 tablespoons ground chia seeds
to 2 dates
cups unsweetened coconut milk
Zest and juice of 1 lime

Directions:
Put all the ingredients in a food processor and pulse until creamy and smooth.
Pour the mixture in a bowl, then wrap in plastic. Store in the refrigerator for at least 20 minutes, then serve chilled.

Per Serving:
calories: 225 | fat: 20.1g | protein: 3.2g | carbs: 5.9g | fiber: 5.0g | sodium: 314mg

Honey Baked Cinnamon Apples

Prep time: 5 minutes | Cook time: 20 minutes | Serves 2

Ingredients:

1 teaspoon extra-virgin olive oil

4 firm apples, peeled, cored, and sliced

½ teaspoon salt

1½ teaspoons ground cinnamon, divided

2 tablespoons unsweetened almond milk

2 tablespoons honey

Directions:

Preheat the oven to 375°F (190°C). Coat a small casserole dish with the olive oil.

Toss the apple slices with the salt and ½ teaspoon of the cinnamon in a medium bowl. Spread the apples in the prepared casserole dish and bake in the preheated oven for 20 minutes.

Meanwhile, in a small saucepan, heat the milk, honey, and remaining 1 teaspoon of cinnamon over medium heat, stirring frequently.

When it reaches a simmer, remove the pan from the heat and cover to keep warm.

Divide the apple slices between 2 plates and pour the sauce over the apples. Serve warm.

Per Serving:

calories: 310 | fat: 3.4g | protein: 1.7g | carbs: 68.5g | fiber: 12.6g | sodium: 593mg

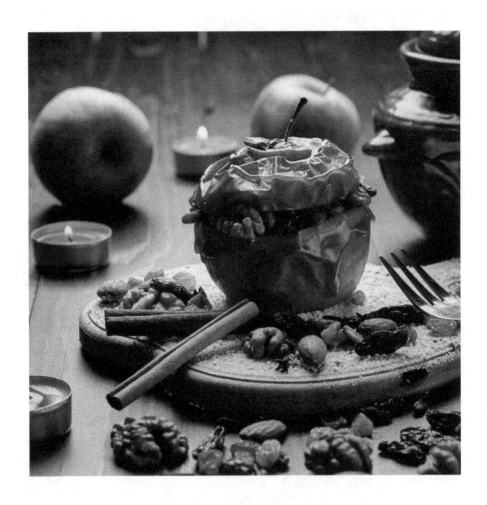

Strawberries with Balsamic Vinegar

Prep time: 5 minutes | Cook time: 0 minutes | Serves 2

Ingredients:
2 cups strawberries, hulled and sliced
2 tablespoons sugar
2 tablespoons balsamic vinegar

Directions:
Place the sliced strawberries in a bowl, sprinkle with the sugar, and drizzle lightly with the balsamic vinegar.
Toss to combine well and allow to sit for about 10 minutes before serving.

Per Serving:
calories: 92 | fat: 0.4g | protein: 1.0g | carbs: 21.7g | fiber: 2.9g | sodium: 5mg

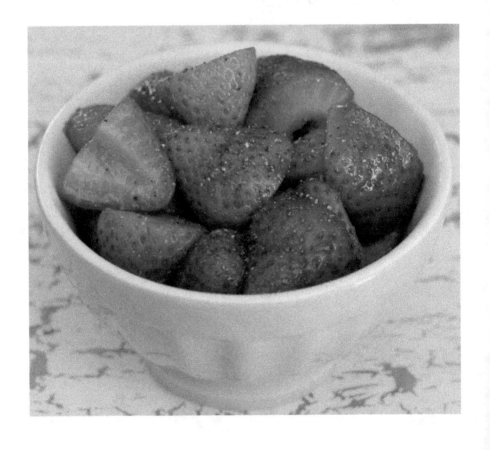

Banana, Cranberry, and Oat Bars

Prep time: 15 minutes | Cook time: 40 minutes | Makes 16 bars

Ingredients:
2 tablespoon extra-virgin olive oil
2 medium ripe bananas, mashed
½ cup almond butter
½ cup maple syrup
⅓ cup dried cranberries
1½ cups old-fashioned rolled oats
¼ cup oat flour
¼ cup ground flaxseed
¼ teaspoon ground cloves
½ cup shredded coconut
½ teaspoon ground cinnamon
1 teaspoon vanilla extract

Directions:
Preheat the oven to 400°F (205°C). Line a 8-inch square pan with parchment paper, then grease with olive oil.
Combine the mashed bananas, almond butter, and maple syrup in a bowl. Stir to mix well.
Mix in the remaining ingredients and stir to mix well until thick and sticky.
Spread the mixture evenly on the square pan with a spatula, then bake in the preheated oven for 40 minutes or until a toothpick inserted in the center comes out clean.
Remove them from the oven and slice into 16 bars to serve.

Per Serving:
calories: 145 | fat: 7.2g | protein: 3.1g | carbs: 18.9g | fiber: 2.0g | sodium: 3m

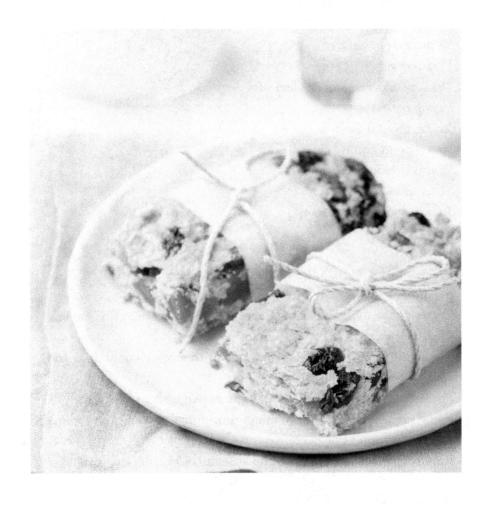

Sauces, Dips, and Dressings

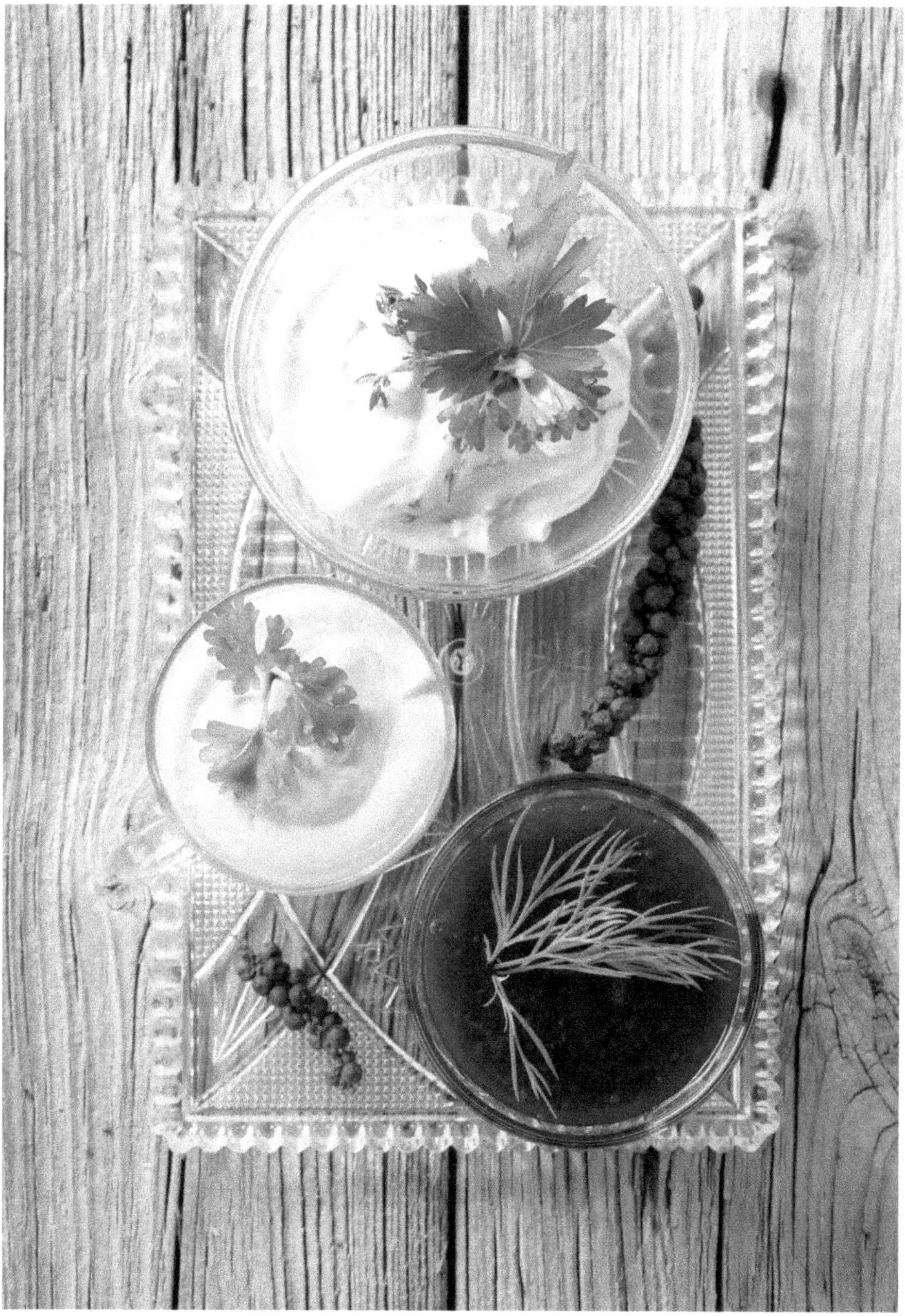

Ranch-Style Cauliflower Dressing

Prep time: 10 minutes | Cook time: 0 minutes | Serves 8

Ingredients:
2 cups frozen cauliflower, thawed
½ cup unsweetened plain almond milk
2 tablespoons apple cider vinegar
2 tablespoons extra-virgin olive oil
garlic clove, peeled
teaspoons finely chopped fresh parsley
2 teaspoons finely chopped scallions (both white and green parts)
1 teaspoon finely chopped fresh dill
½ teaspoon onion powder
½ teaspoon Dijon mustard
½ teaspoon salt
¼ teaspoon freshly ground black pepper

Directions:
Place all the ingredients in a blender and pulse until creamy and smooth.
Serve immediately, or transfer to an airtight container to refrigerate for up to 3 days.

Per Serving: (2 tablespoons)
calories: 41 | fat: 3.6g | protein: 1.0g | carbs: 1.9g | fiber: 1.1g | sodium: 148mg

Asian-Inspired Vinaigrette

Prep time: 5 minutes | Cook time: 0 minutes | Serves 2

Ingredients:
¼ cup extra-virgin olive oil
3 tablespoons apple cider vinegar
1 garlic clove, minced
1 tablespoon peeled and grated fresh ginger
1 tablespoon chopped fresh cilantro
1 tablespoon freshly squeezed lime juice
½ teaspoon sriracha

Directions:
Add all the ingredients in a small bowl and stir to mix well.
Serve immediately, or store covered in the refrigerator and shake before using.

Per Serving:
calories: 251 | fat: 26.8g | protein: 0g | carbs: 1.8g | fiber: 0.7g | sodium: 3mg

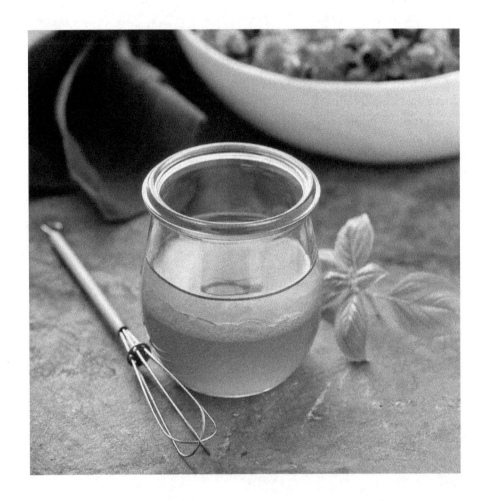

Garlic Lemon-Tahini Dressing

Prep time: 5 minutes | Cook time: 0 minutes | Serves 8 to 10

Ingredients:
½ cup tahini
¼ cup extra-virgin olive oil
¼ cup freshly squeezed lemon juice
garlic clove, finely minced
teaspoons salt

Directions:
In a glass mason jar with a lid, combine the tahini, olive oil, lemon juice, garlic, and salt. Cover and shake well until combined and creamy. Store in the refrigerator for up to 2 weeks.

Per Serving:
calories: 121 | fat: 12.0g | protein: 2.0g | carbs: 3.0g | fiber: 1.0g | sodium: 479mg

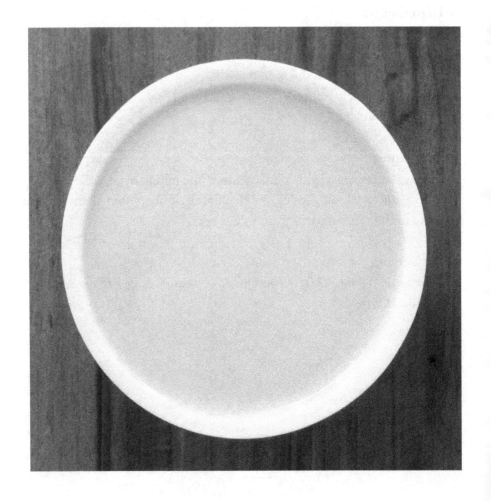

Creamy Grapefruit and Tarragon Dressing

Prep time: 5 minutes | Cook time: 0 minutes | Serves 4 to 6

Ingredients:
½ cup avocado oil mayonnaise
2 tablespoons Dijon mustard
1 teaspoon dried tarragon or 1 tablespoon chopped fresh tarragon
½ teaspoon salt
Zest and juice of ½ grapefruit
¼ teaspoon freshly ground black pepper
1 to 2 tablespoons water (optional)

Directions:
In a large mason jar with a lid, combine the mayonnaise, Dijon, tarragon, grapefruit zest and juice, salt, and pepper and whisk well with a fork until smooth and creamy. If a thinner dressing is preferred, thin out with water.
Serve immediately or refrigerate until ready to serve.

Per Serving:
calories: 86 | fat: 7.0g | protein: 1.0g | carbs: 6.0g | fiber: 0g | sodium: 390mg

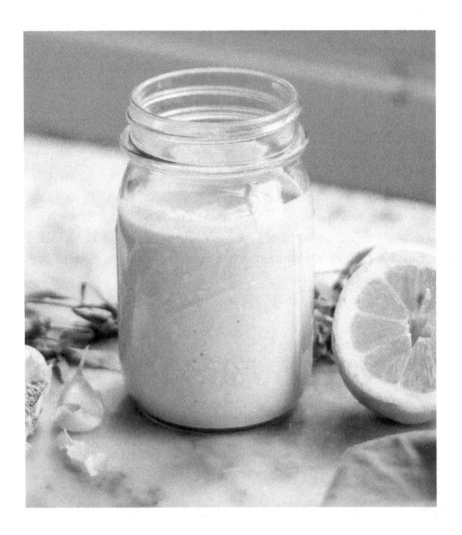

Peri-Peri Sauce

Prep time: 10 minutes | Cook time: 5 minutes | Serves 4

Ingredients:
1 tomato, chopped
1 red onion, chopped
1 red bell pepper, deseeded and chopped
1 red chile, deseeded and chopped
4 garlic cloves, minced
2 tablespoons extra-virgin olive oil
Juice of 1 lemon
1 tablespoon dried oregano
1 tablespoon smoked paprika
1 teaspoon sea salt

Directions:
Process all the ingredients in a food processor or a blender until smooth.

Transfer the mixture to a small saucepan over medium-high heat and bring to a boil, stirring often.

Reduce the heat to medium and allow to simmer for 5 minutes until heated through.

You can store the sauce in an airtight container in the refrigerator for up to 5 days.

Per Serving:
calories: 98 | fat: 6.5g | protein: 1.0g | carbs: 7.8g | fiber: 3.0g | sodium: 295mg

Other Mediterranean Recipes

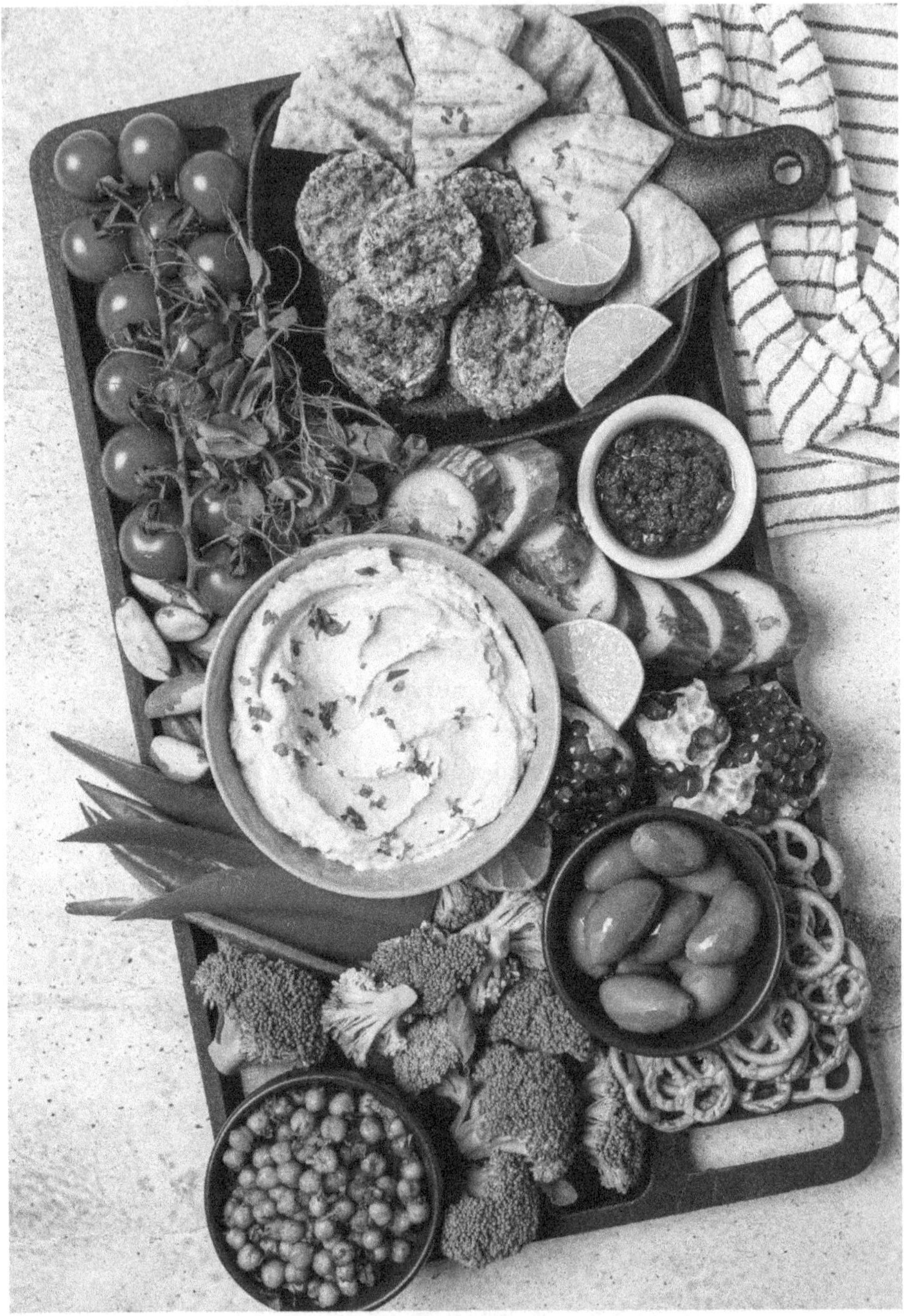

Cauliflower and Sweet Potato

Prep time: 15 minutes | Cook time: 8 minutes | Serves 8

Ingredients:
1 small onion
4 tomatoes
4 garlic cloves, chopped
2-inch ginger, chopped
2 teaspoons olive oil
teaspoon turmeric
teaspoons ground cumin
Salt, to taste
teaspoon paprika
medium sweet potatoes, cubed small
2 small cauliflowers, diced
2 tablespoons fresh cilantro for topping, chopped

Directions:
Blend the tomatoes, garlic, ginger and onion in a blender.
Add the oil and cumin in the instant pot and Sauté for 1 minute.
Stir in the blended mixture and the remaining spices.
Add the sweet potatoes and cook for 5 minutes on Sauté
Add the cauliflower chunks and secure the lid.
Cook on Manual for 2 minutes at High Pressure.
Once done, Quick release the pressure and remove the lid.
Stir and serve with cilantro on top.

Per Serving:
calories: 76 | fat: 1.6g | protein: 2.7g | carbs: 14.4g | fiber: 3.4g | sodium: 55mg

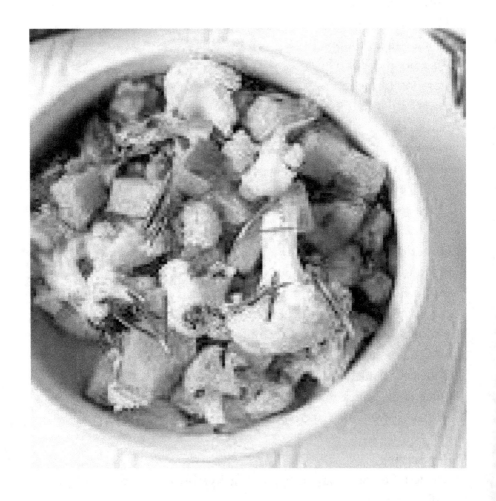

Potato Curry

Prep time: 10 minutes | Cook time: 30 minutes | Serves 2

Ingredients:

2 large potatoes, peeled and diced
1 small onion, peeled and diced
8 ounces (227 g) fresh tomatoes
1 tablespoon olive oil
cup water
tablespoons garlic cloves, grated
½ tablespoon rosemary
½ tablespoon cayenne pepper
1½ tablespoons thyme
Salt and pepper, to taste

Directions:

Pour a cup of water into the instant pot and place the steamer trivet inside.
Place the potatoes and half the garlic over the trivet and sprinkle some salt and pepper on top.
Secure the lid and cook on Steam function for 20 minutes.
After the beep, natural release the pressure and remove the lid.
Put the potatoes to one side and empty the pot.
Add the remaining ingredients to the cooker and Sauté for 10 minutes.
Use an immerse blender to purée the cooked mixture.
Stir in the steamed potatoes and serve hot.

Per Serving:

calories: 398 | fat: 7.6g | protein: 9.6g | carbs: 76.2g | fiber: 10.9g | sodium: 111mg

Veggie Chili

Prep time: 15 minutes | Cook time: 10 minutes | Serves 3

Ingredients:
½ tablespoon olive oil
1 small yellow onion, chopped
4 garlic cloves, minced
¾ (15-ounce / 425-g) can diced tomatoes
1 ounce (28 g) sugar-free tomato paste
½ (4-ounce / 113-g) can green chilies with liquid
tablespoon Worcestershire sauce
tablespoons red chili powder
½ cup carrots, diced
½ cup scallions, chopped
½ cup green bell pepper, chopped
¼ cup peas
1 tablespoon ground cumin
½ tablespoon dried oregano, crushed
Salt and freshly ground black pepper to taste

Directions:
Add the oil, onion, and garlic into the instant pot and Sauté for 5 minutes.
Stir in the remaining vegetables and stir-fry for 3 minutes.
Add the remaining ingredients and secure the lid.
Cook on Manual function for 2 minutes at High Pressure.
After the beep, natural release the pressure and remove the lid.
Stir well and serve warm.

Per Serving:
calories: 106 | fat: 3.9g | protein: 3.4g | carbs: 18.0g | fiber: 6.2g | sodium: 492mg

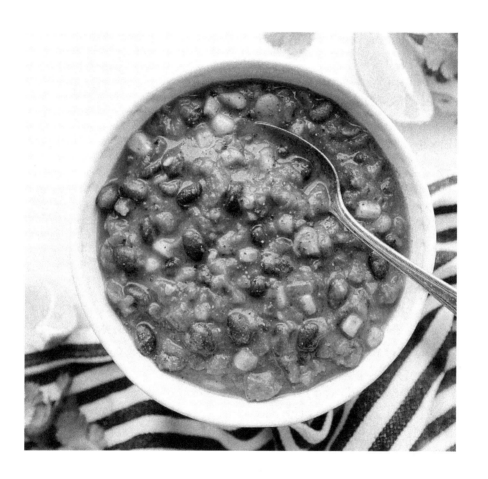

Spiced Citrus Sole

Prep time: 10 minutes | Cook time: 10 minutes | Serves 4

Ingredients:
1 teaspoon garlic powder
1 teaspoon chili powder
½ teaspoon lemon zest
½ teaspoon lime zest
¼ teaspoon smoked paprika
¼ teaspoon freshly ground black pepper
Pinch sea salt
4 (6-ounce / 170-g) sole fillets, patted dry
tablespoon extra-virgin olive oil
teaspoons freshly squeezed lime juice

Directions:
Preheat the oven to 450°F (235°C). Line a baking sheet with aluminum foil and set aside.
Mix together the garlic powder, chili powder, lemon zest, lime zest, paprika, pepper, and salt in a small bowl until well combined.
Arrange the sole fillets on the prepared baking sheet and rub the spice mixture all over the fillets until well coated. Drizzle the olive oil and lime juice over the fillets.
Bake in the preheated oven for about 8 minutes until flaky.
Remove from the heat to a plate and serve.

Per Serving:
calories: 183 | fat: 5.0g | protein: 32.1g | carbs: 0g | fiber: 0g | sodium: 136mg

Crispy Tilapia with Mango Salsa

Prep time: 5 minutes | Cook time: 10 minutes | Serves 2

Ingredients:
Salsa:
cup chopped mango
tablespoons chopped fresh cilantro
2 tablespoons chopped red onion
2 tablespoons freshly squeezed lime juice
½ jalapeño pepper, seeded and minced
Pinch salt
Tilapia:
1 tablespoon paprika
teaspoon onion powder
½ teaspoon dried thyme
½ teaspoon freshly ground black pepper
¼ teaspoon cayenne pepper
½ teaspoon garlic powder
¼ teaspoon salt
½ pound (227 g) boneless tilapia fillets
teaspoons extra-virgin olive oil
1 lime, cut into wedges, for serving

Directions:

Make the salsa: Place the mango, cilantro, onion, lime juice, jalapeño, and salt in a medium bowl and toss to combine. Set aside.

Make the tilapia: Stir together the paprika, onion powder, thyme, black pepper, cayenne pepper, garlic powder, and salt in a small bowl until well mixed. Rub both sides of fillets generously with the mixture.

Heat the olive oil in a large skillet over medium heat.

Add the fish fillets and cook each side for 3 to 5 minutes until golden brown and cooked through.

Divide the fillets among two plates and spoon half of the prepared salsa onto each fillet. Serve the fish alongside the lime wedges.

Per Serving:

calories: 239 | fat: 7.8g | protein: 25.0g | carbs: 21.9g | fiber: 4.0g | sodium: 416mg

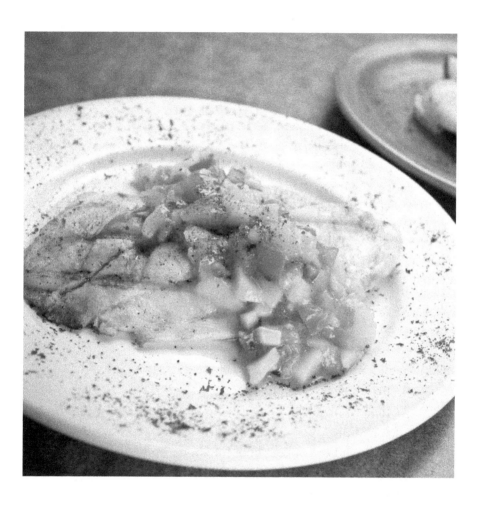

Garlic-Butter Parmesan Salmon and Asparagus

Prep time: 10 minutes | Cook time: 15 minutes | Serves 2

Ingredients:
2 (6-ounce / 170-g) salmon fillets, skin on and patted dry
Pink Himalayan salt
Freshly ground black pepper, to taste
1 pound (454 g) fresh asparagus, ends snapped off
3 tablespoons almond butter
2 garlic cloves, minced
¼ cup grated Parmesan cheese

Directions:
Preheat the oven to 400°F (205°C). Line a baking sheet with aluminum foil.
Season both sides of the salmon fillets with salt and pepper.
Put the salmon in the middle of the baking sheet and arrange the asparagus around the salmon.
Heat the almond butter in a small saucepan over medium heat.
Add the minced garlic and cook for about 3 minutes, or until the garlic just begins to brown.
Drizzle the garlic-butter sauce over the salmon and asparagus and scatter the Parmesan cheese on top.
Bake in the preheated oven for about 12 minutes, or until the salmon is cooked through and the asparagus is crisp-tender. You can switch the oven to broil at the end of cooking time for about 3 minutes to get a nice char on the asparagus.
Let cool for 5 minutes before serving.

Per Serving:
calories: 435 | fat: 26.1g | protein: 42.3g | carbs: 10.0g | fiber: 5.0g | sodium: 503mg

Minestrone Chickpeas and Macaroni Casserole

Prep time: 20 minutes | Cook time: 7 hours 20 minutes | Serves 5

Ingredients:

1 (15-ounce / 425-g) can chickpeas, drained and rinsed
1 (28-ounce / 794-g) can diced tomatoes, with the juice
1 (6-ounce / 170-g) can no-salt-added tomato paste
3 medium carrots, sliced
3 cloves garlic, minced
1 medium yellow onion, chopped
1 cup low-sodium vegetable soup
½ teaspoon dried rosemary
teaspoon dried oregano
teaspoons maple syrup
½ teaspoon sea salt
¼ teaspoon ground black pepper
½ pound (227-g) fresh green beans, trimmed and cut into bite-size pieces
cup macaroni pasta
ounces (57 g) Parmesan cheese, grated

Directions:

Except for the green beans, pasta, and Parmesan cheese, combine all the ingredients in the slow cooker and stir to mix well.
Put the slow cooker lid on and cook on low for 7 hours.
Fold in the pasta and green beans. Put the lid on and cook on high for 20 minutes or until the vegetable are soft and the pasta is al dente.
Pour them in a large serving bowl and spread with Parmesan cheese before serving.

Per Serving:

calories: 349 | fat: 6.7g | protein: 16.5g | carbs: 59.9g | fiber: 12.9g | sodium: 937mg

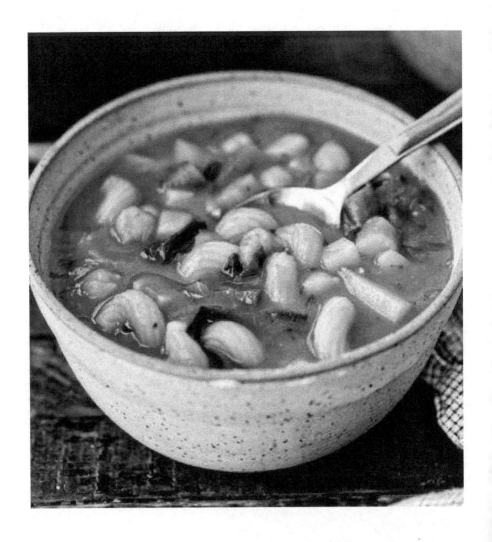

Butternut Squash, Spinach, and Cheeses Lasagna

Prep time: 30 minutes | Cook time: 3 hours 45 minutes | Serves 4 to 6

Ingredients:
2 tablespoons extra-virgin olive oil, divided
butternut squash, halved lengthwise and deseeded
½ teaspoon sage
½ teaspoon sea salt
¼ teaspoon ground black pepper
¼ cup grated Parmesan cheese
cups ricotta cheese
½ cup unsweetened almond milk
5 layers whole-wheat lasagna noodles (about 12 ounces / 340 g in total)
4 ounces (113 g) fresh spinach leaves, divided
½ cup shredded part skim Mozzarella, for garnish

Directions:

Preheat the oven to 400°F (205°C). Line a baking sheet with parchment paper.

Brush 1 tablespoon of olive oil on the cut side of the butternut squash, then place the squash on the baking sheet.

Bake in the preheated oven for 45 minutes or until the squash is tender. Allow to cool until you can handle it, then scoop the flesh out and put the flesh in a food processor to purée.

Combine the puréed butternut squash flesh with sage, salt, and ground black pepper in a large bowl. Stir to mix well.

Combine the cheeses and milk in a separate bowl, then sprinkle with salt and pepper, to taste.

Grease the slow cooker with 1 tablespoon of olive oil, then add a layer of lasagna noodles to coat the bottom of the slow cooker.

Spread half of the squash mixture on top of the noodles, then top the squash mixture with another layer of lasagna noodles.

Spread half of the spinach over the noodles, then top the spinach with half of cheese mixture. Repeat with remaining 3 layers of lasagna noodles, squash mixture, spinach, and cheese mixture.

Top the cheese mixture with Mozzarella, then put the lid on and cook on low for 3 hours or until the lasagna noodles are al dente.

Serve immediately.

Per Serving:

calories: 657 | fat: 37.1g | protein: 30.9g | carbs: 57.2g | fiber: 8.3g | sodium: 918mg

Rich Cauliflower Alfredo

Prep time: 35 minutes | Cook time: 30 minutes | Serves 4

Ingredients:
Cauliflower Alfredo Sauce:
tablespoon avocado oil
½ yellow onion, diced
cups cauliflower florets
2 garlic cloves, minced
1½ teaspoons miso
teaspoon Dijon mustard
Pinch of ground nutmeg
½ cup unsweetened almond milk
1½ tablespoons fresh lemon juice
tablespoons nutritional yeast
Sea salt and ground black pepper, to taste Fettuccine:
1 tablespoon avocado oil
½ yellow onion, diced
1 cup broccoli florets
1 zucchini, halved lengthwise and cut into ¼-inch-thick half-moons
Sea salt and ground black pepper, to taste
½ cup sun-dried tomatoes, drained if packed in oil
8 ounces (227 g) cooked whole-wheat fettuccine
½ cup fresh basil, cut into ribbons

Make the Sauce
Heat the avocado oil in a nonstick skillet over medium-high heat until shimmering.
Add half of the onion to the skillet and sauté for 5 minutes or until translucent.
Add the cauliflower and garlic to the skillet. Reduce the heat to low and cook for 8 minutes or until the cauliflower is tender.
Pour them in a food processor, add the remaining ingredients for the sauce and pulse to combine well. Set aside.

Make the Fettuccine

Heat the avocado oil in a nonstick skillet over medium-high heat. Add the remaining half of onion and sauté for 5 minutes or until translucent.

Add the broccoli and zucchini. Sprinkle with salt and ground black pepper, then sauté for 5 minutes or until tender.

Add the sun-dried tomatoes, reserved sauce, and fettuccine. Sauté for 3 minutes or until well-coated and heated through.

Serve the fettuccine on a large plate and spread with basil before serving.

Per Serving:

calories: 288 | fat: 15.9g | protein: 10.1g | carbs: 32.5g | fiber: 8.1g | sodium: 185mg

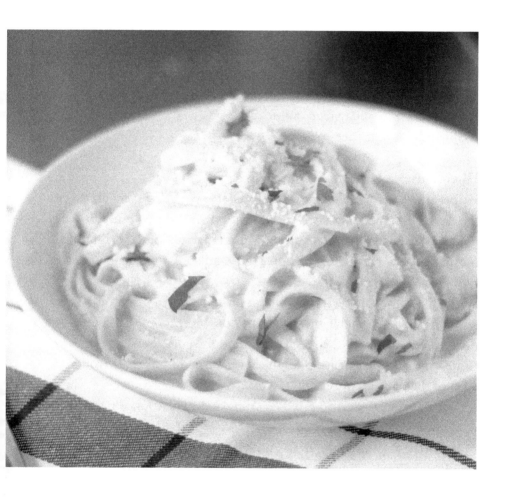

Omelette with Mushrooms and Cheese

Prep time: 30 minutes | Cook time: 15 minutes | Serves 1

Ingredients:
2 eggs
1 teaspoon water (or milk) pinch of kosher salt
1 tablespoon butter (or Cooking spray)
3 brown mushrooms , sliced
5 asparagus spears , trimmed and cut into 1/2-inch pieces
1 tablespoon chopped green onion
2 tablespoons goat cheese

Directions:
Preheat the oven or toaster oven to broil.

Spray a 7- to 8-inch non-stick fry pan with cooking spray and warm on medium heat. Add the sliced mushrooms and cook for 2-3 minutes, turning once or twice. Add the asparagus and cook for 1-2 minutes more.

Whisk the eggs in a bowl with 1 teaspoon water and a pinch of kosher salt until light and frothy, then pour into the mushroom and spinach mixture. Sprinkle with the green onion and the goat cheese.

Cook the eggs undisturbed until the edges begin to pull away from the edge of the pan and begin to set. Gently lift the edges of the egg whites and tilt the pan so the uncooked egg runs under the cooked part and cook for another minute or so.

Transfer the fry pan to the oven and broil for 2-3 minutes or until the eggs have puffed and have cooked through.

Remove from the oven and sprinkle with more goat cheese if desired. Cut into wedges and serve warm or at room temperature.

Per Serving:
calories: 331 | fat: 37.1g | protein: 20g | carbs: 7g | fiber: 2g | sodium: 334mg

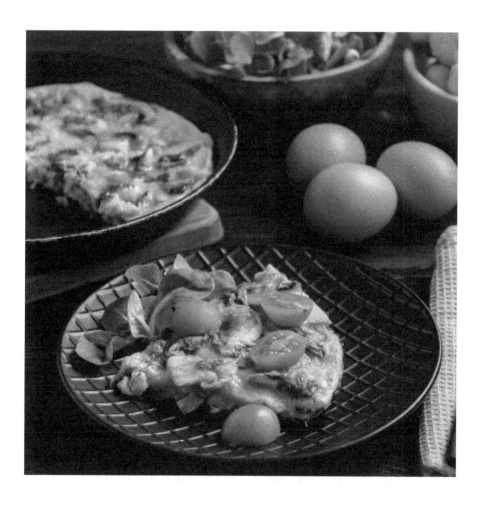

Citrus Shrimp and Avocado Salad

Prep time: 15 minutes | Cook time: 15 minutes | Serves 4

Ingredients:
1 pound medium Pan-Seared Citrus Shrimp (I use 31/40 shrimp)
8 cups greens (such as arugula, spinach, or spring mix)
Fruity or lemon-flavored extra virgin olive oil
Juice of 1/2 lemon or 1/2 orange
1 avocado , sliced or diced
1 shallot , minced
4 ounces sliced almonds , toasted
Kosher salt and freshly ground black pepper

Directions:
Prepare the recipe for the Pan-Seared Citrus Shrimp, or gently warm
the leftover shrimp. Or, if you prefer, serve the shrimp chilled.
Toss the shrimp with the salad greens in a large bowl.
Lightly drizzle with olive oil, and if desired, some of the sauce
remaining from the shrimp with a generous squeeze of citrus, and toss
lightly to coat.
Add the avocado, shallots and sliced almonds and then season with
kosher salt and freshly ground black pepper and serve.

Notes
Use some of the citrus sauce from the shrimp as a double duty
dressing.
Or, if you don't have enough sauce for the dressing, simply use a good
extra virgin olive oil (I like the lemon flavored varieties) with an
additional squeeze of citrus.

Per Serving:
calories: 374 | fat: 23g | protein: 31g | carbs: 14g | fiber: 7g |
sodium: 906mg

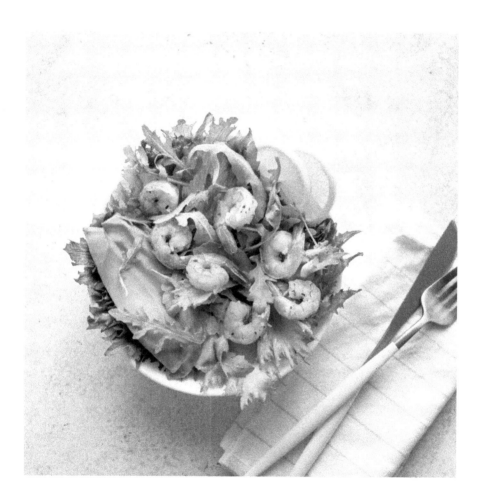

CPSIA information can be obtained
at www.ICGtesting.com
Printed in the USA
BVHW040521190621
609641BV00021B/2946